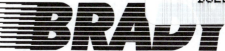

DRUG
DOSAGE
CALCULATIONS

For the Emergency Care Provider

Second Edition

ALAN A. MIKOLAJ, B.S.
Licensed Paramedic

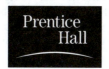

Prentice Hall

Upper Saddle River, New Jersey 07458

Library of Congress Cataloging-in-Publication Data

Mikolaj, Alan A., (date)
  Drug dosage calculations : for the emergency care
    provider / Alan A. Mikolaj.
    p. cm.
  Includes bibliographical references and index.
  ISBN 0–13–091285–9
    1. Pharmaceutical arithmetic. 2. Emergency
  medicine—Mathematics. I. Title: At head of title:
  Brady. II. Title: Drug dosage calculations for the
  emergency care provider. III. Title.

RS57 .M54 2002
615′.14—dc21   2001056784
                                                     CIP

Publisher: *Julie Levin Alexander*
Assistant to Publisher: *Regina Bruno*
Acquisitions Editor: *Katrin Beacom*
Editorial Assistant: *Kierra Kashickey*
Marketing Manager: *Tiffany Price*
Director of Production and Manufacturing:
  Bruce Johnson
Managing Production Editor: *Patrick Walsh*
Manufacturing Buyer: *Pat Brown*
Production Liaison: *Julie Li*
Production Editor: *Pat McCutcheon*
Creative Director: *Cheryl Asherman*
Cover Design Coordinator: *Maria Guglielmo*
Cover Designer: *Gary J. Sella*
Composition: *WestWords, Inc.*
Printing and Binding: *Von Hoffman Press*

Pearson Education LTD.
Pearson Education Australia PTY, Limited
Pearson Education Singapore, Pte. Ltd
Pearson Education North Asia Ltd
Pearson Education Canada, Ltd.
Pearson Educación de Mexico, S.A. de C.V.
Pearson Education—Japan
Pearson Education Malaysia, Pte. Ltd
Pearson Education, Upper Saddle River, New Jersey

Notice: The author and the publisher of this book have taken care to make certain that the equipment, doses of drugs and schedules of treatment are correct and compatible with the standards generally accepted at the time of publication. Nevertheless, as new information becomes available, changes in treatment and in the use of equipment and drugs become necessary. The reader is advised to carefully consult the instruction and information material included in the package insert of each drug or therapeutic agent, piece of equipment or device before administration. This advice is especially important when using new or infrequently used drugs. No endorsement by the American Heart Association or any of its committees is stated or implied, nor is there any suggested warranty of performance during the American Heart Association Advanced Cardiac Life Support Course. Prehospital Care Providers are warned that use of any drugs or techniques must be authorized by their medical advisor, in accord with the local laws and regulations. The publisher disclaims any liability, loss, injury, or damage incurred as a consequence, directly or indirectly, of the use and application of any of the contents of this book.

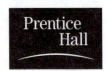

10 9 8 7 6 5 4 3
ISBN 0-13-091285-9

Dedication

For Mom
It's because of you that I do what I do!

Special thanks to:

Joseph E. Peters, Jr., B.S., NREMT-P; William E. Butler, B.S., NREMT-P; the faculty and staff of the University of Texas Health Science Center at San Antonio, Emergency Medical Technology Department for all your tolerance and bolstering support.

And to all my students who helped teach me to be a better instructor and who edited and endured so many trials and errors while I wrote this book.

Contents

Contents   **vii**

Preface

There continues to be a need for a dosage calculations textbook written specifically for emergency care providers, especially prehospital care providers. Because of the expanding nature of the curriculum in prehospital and emergency medicine, most textbooks simply don't have the space necessary to cover the subject in any detail. Many students (and even some faculty) enter the classroom, and unfortunately sometimes into practice, needing an additional resource when it comes to dosage calculations.

This second edition retains the heart of the first: a simple, step-by-step approach focusing on explanation and understanding, organization, and accuracy. While working in the field and in the classroom, I have noticed three distinct areas that pose consistent challenges to both students and practicing emergency health care providers (EMS personnel, nurses, ER physicians, etc.). Those three areas constitute the three sections of Drug Dosage Calculations for the Emergency Care Provider: (1) Mathematics and Fractions Review, (2) Systems of Measurement, and (3) Emergency Drug Dosage Calculations. Not all students require help or instruction in all three areas. Some students may only need instruction or review in one or two areas. Other students may need partial review or instruction in specific sections of all three areas. Still, there are others who will need comprehensive review or instruction in all three areas. Today's adult education and continuing education must take these types of issues into account in order to be successful. This small book was designed to meet those needs. It can stand alone as a continuing education course or be incorporated into existing programs as a supplementary text.

Drug Dosage Calculations for the Emergency Care Provider was written for a special group of people who dedicate themselves to the service of emergency patients. Section One focuses on fractions and basic algebra functions essential to understanding and solving drug dosage calculations. Many students of all ages and careers have used this section to brush up on fractions, decimals, percentages, and basic math skills. Section Two explains the history of systems of measurement, reviews the old customary system, and provides a complete explanation of the metric system and the federally approved rules governing the metric system in the United States. It then describes different techniques for converting between systems. Section Three explains each type of dosage calculation problem that may be encountered in the emergency setting in detail with each chapter providing the building blocks for the next. Alternate techniques/methods of solving problems are presented to accommodate the diversified backgrounds of emergency health care professionals. There are plenty of practical problems that complement emergency pharmacology and prepare the student for practical application.

The second edition has been updated with the addition of new drugs and dosages in practice and test problems. Expanded exercises offer more practice for the student. Refinements in explanation and organization can be found throughout the text. With its simple, easy-to-read format and practical approach, Drug Dosage Calculations for the Emergency Care Provider will make an outstanding addition to your emergency health care training.

I would like to extend special recognition and my sincerest appreciation to the following individuals who served as reviewers. Their scrutiny, suggestions, and support are greatly valued!

Rhonda J. Beck, NREMT-P
Central Georgia Technical College
Houston Medical Center EMS
Macon, Georgia

Jeffery L. Beinke, BS, REMT-P
Division Chair, Allied Health
Technology
Montgomery Community College
Troy, NC

Jim Holbrook, MA, EMT-P
Crafton Hills College
Yucaipa, CA

William Kenney, EMT-P
Medi Flight Oklahoma
Oklahoma City, OK

Mark J. Reis, NREMT-P
State EMS Instructor
Operations Manager, Acadian
Ambulance Service
Covington, LA

Alan A. Mikolaj, B.S.
Licensed Paramedic

Note to Instructors

Prehospital EMS education students are an amazingly diversified group. These very special people come from diverse backgrounds and have a variety of educational histories. Meeting educational objectives with these students can sometimes pose a challenge to the instructor. This becomes especially evident when trying to teach drug dosage calculations. In addition, different programs have different learning objectives. Some require more, others less. Drug Dosage Calculations for the Emergency Care Provider addresses these needs.

While working in the field and in the classroom, I have noticed three distinct areas that consistently pose challenges to both students and practicing emergency health care providers. This text is divided into three sections addressing each of those areas:

- Section One: Mathematics and Fractions Review
- Section Two: Systems of Measurement
- Section Three: Drug Dosage Calculations

Not all students will need intensive instruction in all three areas. Using this text does not necessarily demand that you use the entirety of each of the three sections in your classroom/lecture time. You may only need to use parts of sections or spend considerably less time on some of them. Curriculum and lesson plans must be tailored to meet the needs of the students and the program in order to be successful. Sometimes, individual tutoring or special sessions for those students who necessitate more intensive remedial work can be incorporated into existing programs. However, I have found that all students have something to gain or contribute when incorporating all three sections into drug dosage calculation instruction. Other instructor and student feedback confirms this.

Feel free to utilize the text to fit your needs. There are going to be some students that require some level of remedial instruction and practice in Section One and/or Two before being able to engage in the work required by Section Three. The first two sections are provided to meet those needs. I have tried various methods with various student populations, Department of Defense Special Operations Forces, municipal and rural fire departments and EMS groups (both paid and volunteer), and initial and continuing education groups. Encouraging the more advanced students to work with remedial students during review of Sections One and Two via a variety of teaching techniques seems to facilitate the learning process for both groups of students. Your students will determine how much time and effort is required in each of these areas.

This is one of the more difficult parts of the curriculum to both teach and learn. Hats off to you for taking on this task! Your level of enthusiasm and effort for any subject matter will have an impact on your students' enthusiasm and effort. It is my sincere intent that this text makes that easier for you and your students.

Alan

About the Author

Alan A. Mikolaj, B.S. received his introduction to prehospital care from his mother. She volunteered as an EMT-I for the Timber Lakes Volunteer Fire Department near Houston, Texas. It was watching her (and listening to her stories) that prompted him to take a position in 1979 as an emergency dispatcher for the Woodlands Fire Department and South Montgomery County. In 1982 he received his Emergency Medical Technician training through the Montgomery County Hospital District and the Timber Lakes Volunteer Fire Department. He has served in the U.S. Army as a combat medic/Battalion Aid Station non-commissioned officer in-charge at Ft. Carson, Colo., in a mechanized infantry unit. As a practical nurse at Brooke Army Medical Center's (BAMC) Female Surgical Orthopedic Ward at Ft. Sam Houston, Texas, Mr. Mikolaj received special experience in the postsurgical clinical environment. While at Ft. Sam Houston, he also held the position of triage specialist in BAMC's emergency room. While in the Army, he attended night school at the University of Texas Health Science Center in San Antonio, earning his paramedic certification. Mr. Mikolaj has worked in all areas of the prehospital care environment. He has worked for locally governed 911/ACLS services, private ambulance services, in the offshore environment, and in the training and educational arenas at both the community college and university levels. He has taught and been preceptor to hundreds of students, both civilian and military. He obtained his bachelor's of science degree in psychology from Sam Houston State University. He is currently enrolled there as a graduate student in the Master of Clinical Psychology Program. Mr. Mikolaj works as a licensed paramedic in the Houston area and volunteers regularly with the Bluebonnet Critical Incident Stress Management organization serving the greater Houston area.

SECTION ONE

MATHEMATICS AND FRACTIONS REVIEW

This section will review the basic math skills required for most dosage calculations. It is divided into easily understood units explaining fractions, decimals, percentages, ratios, and proportions. It provides examples, exercises, and plenty of problems to help hone your mathematical skills.

When we desire to encourage the growth of the human spirit, we challenge and encourage the human capacity to solve problems, just as in school, we deliberately set problems for our children to solve. It is through the pain of confronting and resolving problems that we learn.

—M. Scott Peck L.M.D.—
The Road Less Traveled

Introduction

Today's emergency health care providers require a firm foundation in basic mathematics in order to calculate drug dosages. With advancing prehospital and emergency room care, changes in Advanced Cardiac Life Support standards and guidelines, and the addition of new drugs in emergency care, it becomes essential to perform accurate dosage calculations to ensure that patients receive the correct dosages. Often, these calculations will be performed while managing the critical patients in sometimes severe environments. When faced with a critical situation, you'll be glad you took the time to prepare and become competent in your math skills.

This section reviews the basic math skills required for most dosage calculations. It is divided into easily understood chapters explaining fractions, decimals, percentages, ratios, and proportions. It provides examples and exercises to hone your mathematical skills.

Because prehospital and emergency care students come from such diverse backgrounds and experiences, some individuals require more review and practice than others. The time to find out about your math skills is *now*. If you wait and find out during a complicated explanation of a dosage calculation, you can miss valuable information and waste precious time. To help you determine just how much practice you may need and in which chapters you may need it, the following pretest will assess your knowledge of basic mathematics concepts and your ability to solve common arithmetic problems. The answer key in Appendix A will show you the answers and the chapter where explanations for that problem may be found.

Pretest

Directions: Answer the following questions. Reduce all fractions to their lowest terms. Round decimals to the nearest hundredth. For answers and chapter references, see Appendix A.

In the following fractions identify the denominator:

1. $\dfrac{1}{3}$

2. $\dfrac{9}{7}$

In the following fractions identify the numerator:

3. $\dfrac{1}{3}$

4. $\dfrac{9}{7}$

In the following fractions, identify whether it is a complex fraction, a proper fraction, or an improper fraction:

5. $\dfrac{1/2}{3/4}$

6. $\dfrac{3}{4}$

7. $\dfrac{5}{4}$

Convert the following mixed numbers to improper fractions:

8. $1\dfrac{1}{4}$

9. $10\dfrac{5}{6}$

In the following fractions, convert the improper fractions to mixed numbers:

10. $\dfrac{13}{4}$

11. $\dfrac{97}{9}$

Check the equality of the following fractions:

12. $\dfrac{6}{9} = \dfrac{30}{45}$

13. $\dfrac{12}{13} = \dfrac{60}{67}$

Add the following fractions:

14. $\dfrac{1}{2} + \dfrac{3}{7} + \dfrac{2}{9} =$

15. $7\dfrac{1}{3} + 2\dfrac{2}{5} + 3\dfrac{16}{90} =$

Subtract the following fractions:

16. $\dfrac{1}{8} - \dfrac{1}{12} =$

17. $6\dfrac{2}{3} - 5\dfrac{3}{4} =$

Multiply the following fractions:

18. $1\dfrac{1}{2} \times 2\dfrac{1}{4} =$

19. $\dfrac{1}{2} \times \dfrac{1}{3} \times \dfrac{1}{14} =$

Divide the following fractions:

20. $\dfrac{1}{100} \div \dfrac{2}{3} =$

21. $150\dfrac{3}{4} \div \dfrac{1}{18} =$

Add the following decimals:

22. $10.2 + 32.3 + 1.45 =$

23. $0.0001 + 1.05 + 4.006 + 2 =$

Subtract the following decimals:

24. $2.5 - 0.95 =$

25. $0.912 - 0.099 =$

Multiply the following decimals:

26. $1.5 \times 3.75 =$

27. $0.0033 \times 9.02 =$

Divide the following decimals:

28. $100 \div 3.5 =$

29. $0.625 \div 3.3 =$

Work or solve the following ratio problems:

30. Express $\dfrac{3}{20}$ as a ratio.

31. Express $3:1$ as a common fraction.

32. $6:12::9:X$

33. $\dfrac{5}{15} = \dfrac{6}{X}$

Work the following percent problems:

34. What is 25% of 100?

35. 45 is what percent of 250?

36. 60% of what number is 150?

Convert:

37. $2:3$ to a decimal.

38. 0.25 to a fraction.

39. 0.45 to a percent.

40. 55% to a fraction.

Common Fractions

OBJECTIVES

In order to work dosage calculation problems as an emergency health care provider, you should be able to:

1. Define a fraction.

2. Define and identify the denominator in a fraction.

3. Define and identify the numerator in a fraction.

4. Define and identify a common fraction.

5. Define and identify a complex fraction.

6. Define and identify a proper fraction.

7. Define and identify an improper fraction.

8. Define and identify a mixed number.

9. Convert mixed numbers to improper fractions.

10. Convert improper fractions to mixed numbers.

11. Reduce common fractions to the lowest terms.

12. Identify and utilize fractions as the number one.

13. Find the lowest common denominator of common fractions.

14. Apply the cross-multiplication technique to check the equality of common fractions.

15. Add common fractions.

16. Subtract common fractions.

17. Multiply common fractions.

18. Divide common fractions.

INTRODUCTION

- *Is a denominator the number on the top or on the bottom of a fraction?*
- *What's an improper fraction?*
- *How do you find the lowest common denominator?*
- *What are the steps to divide fractions?*

If these are questions that you could be asking, you may want to spend some time working in this chapter. This chapter reviews common fractions. It will answer all the questions above plus many others. In addition to reviewing common fractions, it will explain the cross-multiplication technique, and review addition, subtraction, multiplication, and division of common fractions. There are plenty of practice problems with answers in the back of the book.

Mathematics, rightly viewed, possesses not only truth,
But supreme beauty—a beauty cold and austere,
Like that of sculpture.
—Bertrand Russell—

1.1 FRACTION FUNDAMENTALS

Since it may have been some time since you last worked with fractions, this preliminary review of fraction fundamentals may prove helpful. A **fraction** is a mathematical representation for parts of a whole. In other words, something has been equally divided. It consists of one number over another separated by a short line. The bottom number, or the **denominator,** represents the total number of equal parts in the whole. The top number, or the **numerator,** represents the number of parts of the whole that are being considered.

For example, in the fraction $\frac{3}{4}$, the 4 is the denominator and signifies four equal parts of the whole (see Figure 1.1). The 3 is the numerator and signifies that only three of the four parts are being considered.

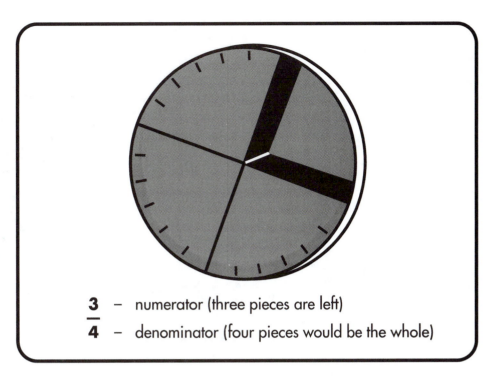

$$\frac{3}{4}$$ – numerator (three pieces are left)
– denominator (four pieces would be the whole)

Figure 1.1 Fractions are parts of the whole.

The fraction $\frac{3}{4}$ can be referred to as a **common fraction.** In a common fraction, the numerator and the denominator are both whole numbers. These are the type of fractions most people think about when fractions are considered. In another type of fraction, a **complex fraction,** the numerator and denominator themselves are fractions, such as

$$\frac{1/4}{3/4}$$

Common fractions can be described as either proper fractions or improper fractions. Sometimes, just parts of one whole are considered. This is called a **proper fraction.** In a proper fraction the numerator is smaller than the denominator, such as with the fraction $\frac{3}{4}$. Sometimes, more than one whole is considered. When this is expressed as a fraction, it is called an **improper fraction** (see Figure 1.2). When more than one whole is being calculated, the numerator will exceed the denominator, such as $\frac{5}{4}$.

An improper fraction can also be described using whole numbers and fractions. When formulated this way, the expression is referred to as a **mixed number.** The fraction $\frac{5}{4}$ in Figure 1.2 could also be expressed as the mixed number $1\frac{1}{4}$.

Mixed Number Conversion

Being able to convert mixed numbers to improper fractions and vice versa will be necessary when calculating drug dosages. This is done quite easily. When faced with a mixed number, multiply the denominator by the whole number and then add the numerator to that sum. To convert the mixed

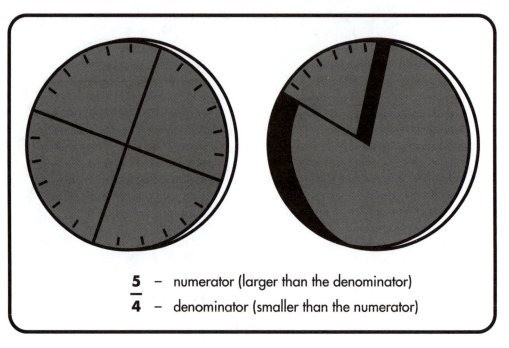

$\dfrac{5}{4}$ – numerator (larger than the denominator)

denominator (smaller than the numerator)

Figure 1.2 Improper fraction.

number $1\frac{1}{4}$ to an improper fraction, for example, multiply the denominator 4 by the whole number 1:

$$1\frac{1}{4}$$

$$4 \times 1 = 4$$

Now, add the numerator 1 to the above sum:

$$4 + 1 = 5$$

The 5 is now the new numerator. The denominator stays the same and the new improper fraction is

$$\frac{5}{4}$$

To convert an improper fraction to a mixed number, just reverse the process. Divide the numerator 5 by the denominator 4 to obtain 1 with a remainder of $\frac{1}{4}$ or $1\frac{1}{4}$.

Reducing to Lowest Terms

Usually, most fractions are reduced to their **lowest terms.** All answers in this book will be reduced to their lowest term, as well. This is also referred to as simplifying a fraction. This can be done two ways.

One way to reduce a fraction to the lowest terms is to determine the largest common divisor of both the numerator and the denominator and divide them both by that number. This will involve some guesswork and may take several attempts.

Another more accurate method is to factor the numerator and the denominator to their prime numbers. (**Prime numbers** are divisible only by

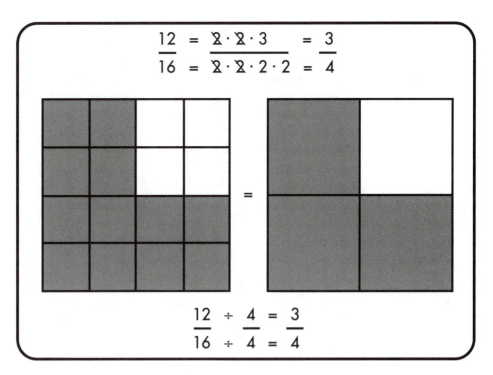

Figure 1.3 Reducing fractions to the lowest terms.

themselves and the number 1. For example, the numbers 1, 2, 3, 5, and 7 are prime numbers.) When this is done, the numbers that repeat in the numerator and the denominator "cancel out." Look at Figure 1.3 to see how to reduce the fraction $\frac{12}{16}$ to the lowest terms.

Fractions as the Number One

As you can see, the fraction $\frac{4}{4}$ was used to reduce the fraction $\frac{12}{16}$ to the fraction $\frac{3}{4}$. A simple rule to remember is: *Any number over itself is the number 1*. If there are $\frac{4}{4}$ of a pie, it means that one whole is divided into four equal parts. The fraction $\frac{12}{16}$ was simply divided by the number 1 in the form of a fraction. When looking at Figure 1.3, the fraction $\frac{12}{16}$ and the fraction $\frac{3}{4}$ are equal. The only difference is that the fraction $\frac{12}{16}$ is divided into more pieces. The concept of fractions as the number 1 proves useful when reducing fractions to their lowest terms or when trying to find the lowest common denominator. Knowing and applying this principle will occasionally be necessary when calculating drug dosage problems.

Lowest Common Denominator

Trying to find the **lowest common denominator** is another tool necessary for working with fractions. You could have a problem involving fractions with different denominators and need common denominators to work your problem. For example, the fractions $\frac{1}{3}$, $\frac{7}{12}$, and $\frac{3}{4}$ need to be used in a problem with the same denominator. You could multiply the denominators by each other and arrive at *a* common denominator:

$$3 \times 12 \times 4 = 144$$

The 144 could be used as a common denominator for all three fractions, and it would then be necessary to convert each fraction to have a denominator of 144. But this may not give you the *lowest* common denominator. A lowest common denominator will be easier to work with than a larger common denominator. Here is one way to find the lowest common denominator.

First, list the denominators in a horizontal row across the chart in Figure 1.4. Then, divide the denominators by prime factors in the vertical column to the left. Start with the smallest prime factor that divides into one of the denominators evenly—in this example, 2. Bring down any numbers that are not evenly divisible by a prime factor to the next row of boxes. Repeat this process until the numbers in the bottom row of boxes cannot be divided any further. If two or more of the same prime factors are left in the bottom row, you must divide out those prime factors.

There should only be prime factors down the vertical column and only prime factors that are not repeated in the horizontal row. Multiply the prime factors in the vertical column by the prime factors left in the horizontal row together to arrive at the lowest common denominator. See Figure 1.4 for an illustration of this method using the fractions $\frac{1}{3}$, $\frac{7}{12}$, and $\frac{3}{4}$. The number 12 is the lowest common denominator.

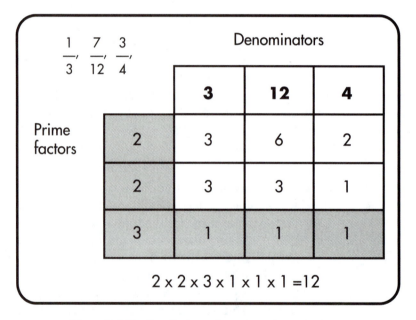

Figure 1.4 Finding the lowest common denominator.

Converting

It is now necessary to convert each of the fractions to fractions with a denominator of 12. Multiply the fractions $\frac{1}{3}$, $\frac{7}{12}$, and $\frac{3}{4}$ by 1 in the form of a fraction that will convert the fractions to have a denominator of 12. Here's how:

1. Take the denominator of the fraction needing conversion and divide it into the lowest common denominator. The quotient becomes the number to use as 1 in the form of a fraction.

2. Multiply the fraction requiring conversion by that number 1 in the form of a fraction. For instance, in the fraction $\frac{1}{3}$, $12 \div 3 = 4$. Use the 4 as the number 1 in the form of a fraction $\left(\frac{4}{4}\right)$ to convert $\frac{1}{3}$ to the fraction $\frac{4}{12}$. Use this technique to convert all the fractions:

$$\frac{1}{3} \times \frac{4}{4} = \frac{4}{12}$$

$$\frac{7}{12} \times \frac{1}{1} = \frac{7}{12}$$

$$\frac{3}{4} \times \frac{3}{3} = \frac{9}{12}$$

They have now been converted to fractions with the lowest common denominator.

Cross-Multiplication

The converted fractions above are equal to the original fractions. This is proved using a concept called **cross-multiplication.** Look at the fraction $\frac{1}{3}$ compared to $\frac{4}{12}$. When the numerators of each fraction are multiplied by the denominators of the other, the products should be equal:

$$\frac{1}{3} = \frac{4}{12}$$

$$1 \times 12 = \mathbf{12}$$

$$3 \times 4 = \mathbf{12}$$

When the products are equal, the fractions are equal. If the products are not equal, the fractions are not equal. Cross-multiplication is a very important technique that will be used later with drug dosage calculations.

Whole Numbers as Fractions

There is another item worth mentioning before we go on. Any whole number not associated with a fraction can be expressed as a fraction. Simply place the whole number as the numerator of a fraction over the denominator of 1. This creates an improper fraction. For example, 3 can be expressed as the fraction

$$\frac{3}{1}$$

Reduction of Numbers Ending in Zero

The last element in this review concerns reductions when both the numerator and the denominator end with zeros. Fractions in which the numerator and denominator both end in a zero or zeros may be reduced by crossing off an equal number of zeros in each. Take, for example, the fraction

$$\frac{250}{1000}$$

The numerator, 250, has one zero at the end, and the denominator, 1000, has three zeros at the end. Because the number 250 only has one zero, only one zero can be crossed off both numbers

$$\frac{25\cancel{0}}{100\cancel{0}} = \frac{25}{100}$$

Now, further reductions or calculations can more easily be performed.

EXERCISE 1.1 FRACTION FUNDAMENTALS

(Answers may be found in Appendix B.)

Identify the numerator in the following fractions:

1. $\dfrac{2}{7}$

2. $\dfrac{5}{16}$

3. $\dfrac{17}{100}$

4. $\dfrac{2}{3}$

5. $\dfrac{4}{7}$

Identify the denominator in the following fractions:

6. $\dfrac{2}{5}$

7. $\dfrac{7}{8}$

8. $\dfrac{29}{35}$

9. $\dfrac{1}{11}$

10. $\dfrac{3}{2}$

Identify the following fractions as either proper or improper:

11. $\dfrac{7}{3}$

12. $\dfrac{3}{4}$

13. $\dfrac{5}{12}$

14. $\dfrac{12}{5}$

15. $\dfrac{2}{5}$

Convert the following improper fractions to mixed numbers:

16. $\dfrac{7}{3}$

17. $\dfrac{19}{6}$

18. $\dfrac{39}{6}$

19. $\dfrac{114}{12}$

20. $\dfrac{50}{18}$

Convert the following mixed numbers to improper fractions:

21. $1\dfrac{1}{2}$

22. $2\dfrac{1}{3}$

23. $16\dfrac{1}{6}$

24. $33\dfrac{1}{3}$

25. $9\dfrac{2}{5}$

Reduce the following fractions to the lowest terms:

26. $\dfrac{25}{100}$

27. $\dfrac{8}{10}$

28. $\dfrac{10}{100}$

29. $\dfrac{19}{76}$

30. $\dfrac{34}{51}$

For the following sets of fractions, find the lowest common denominator and convert:

31. $\dfrac{1}{3}, \dfrac{1}{4}, \dfrac{1}{2}$

32. $\dfrac{1}{2}, \dfrac{1}{8}, \dfrac{1}{16}$

33. $\dfrac{1}{2}, \dfrac{2}{3}, \dfrac{5}{6}, \dfrac{7}{9}$

34. $\dfrac{23}{24}, \dfrac{15}{48}, \dfrac{74}{80}$

35. $\dfrac{1}{9}, \dfrac{11}{24}, \dfrac{7}{18}$

Check the equality of the following fractions:

36. $\dfrac{1}{2} = \dfrac{35}{70}$

37. $\dfrac{4}{5} = \dfrac{32}{40}$

38. $\dfrac{3}{8} = \dfrac{9}{23}$

39. $\dfrac{5}{4} = \dfrac{45}{36}$

40. $\dfrac{9}{7} = \dfrac{36}{35}$

1.2 ADDITION OF FRACTIONS

Someone has divided the volume of a drug one way and someone else has divided the same volume another way. You want to know the total amount of drug that is available. How are fractions with different denominators added? There is an easy three-step method. Look at the following problem as an example:

$$\frac{3}{8} + \frac{1}{12} = ?$$

The two fractions are describing two different wholes that have been divided differently. To add them, they must be compared to equal divisions. This leads us to the first step:

1. **Find the lowest common denominators.** To solve this problem, first find the lowest common denominators using the method described in

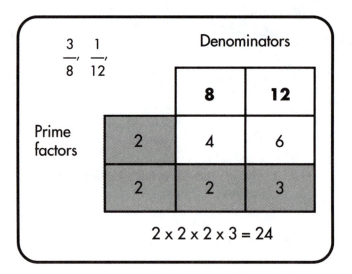

Figure 1.5 Lowest common denominator.

Section 1.1, Fraction Fundamentals (p. 8). Review Figure 1.5 to see how the lowest common denominator was found for the fractions $\frac{3}{8}$ and $\frac{1}{12}$.

2. **Convert the fractions.** Now that the lowest common denominator has been found, it is necessary to multiply the fractions by 1 in the form of a fraction to convert them into fractions with common denominators, (see pages 11–12 for a review of this process in Section 1.1, Fraction Fundamentals):

$$\frac{3}{8} \times \frac{3}{3} = \frac{9}{24}$$

$$\frac{1}{12} \times \frac{2}{2} = \frac{2}{24}$$

3. **Add the numerators.** Now that the fractions have common denominators and they have been converted, the fractions can be added together. Fractions with common denominators are added by adding the *numerators only* and placing the sum over the common denominator. Remember, *reduce if possible*. See the following example:

$$\frac{9}{24} + \frac{2}{24} = \frac{11}{24}$$

NOTE: When faced with mixed numbers, you can *either* add the whole numbers separately and then add them to the sum of the remaining fractions (and reduce) *or* convert the mixed numbers to an improper fraction and add the fractions as above.

(Answers may be found in Appendix B.)

Directions: Add the following fractions and reduce if possible.

1. $\dfrac{2}{5} + \dfrac{1}{5} =$

2. $\dfrac{2}{3} + \dfrac{1}{6} =$

3. $\dfrac{3}{4} + \dfrac{1}{8} + \dfrac{1}{6} =$

4. $3 + 1\dfrac{1}{3} =$

5. $1\dfrac{1}{2} + \dfrac{3}{4} =$

6. $2\dfrac{1}{6} + 3\dfrac{1}{3} =$

7. $\dfrac{1}{2} + \dfrac{1}{6} + 2\dfrac{1}{3} =$

8. $5\dfrac{1}{2} + 2\dfrac{3}{4} =$

9. $\dfrac{1}{2} + \dfrac{2}{3} + \dfrac{5}{6} + 1\dfrac{7}{9} =$

10. $7\dfrac{1}{3} + 2\dfrac{2}{5} + 3\dfrac{16}{90} =$

11. $7\dfrac{1}{8} + 4\dfrac{2}{3} =$

12. $\dfrac{3}{8} + \dfrac{5}{12} + \dfrac{1}{9} =$

13. $1\dfrac{1}{5} + \dfrac{7}{10} + 4\dfrac{1}{3} =$

14. $\dfrac{3}{4} + 6\dfrac{1}{3} + 2\dfrac{5}{14} =$

15. $2\dfrac{7}{12} + \dfrac{5}{8} + 4 =$

1.3 SUBTRACTION OF FRACTIONS

Subtraction of common fractions is a lot like addition of common fractions. If the denominators are not the same, it requires conversion to fractions with common denominators before the function can be carried out. Take a look at the following example:

$$\frac{3}{8} - \frac{1}{12} = ?$$

1. **Find the lowest common denominator.** For the numbers 8 and 12, the lowest common denominator is 24.

2. **Convert the fractions.** Multiply the fractions by the number 1 in the form of a fraction after the lowest common denominator has been determined.

$$\frac{3}{8} \times \frac{3}{3} = \frac{9}{24}$$

$$\frac{1}{12} \times \frac{2}{2} = \frac{2}{24}$$

$$\frac{3}{8} = \frac{9}{24}$$

$$\frac{1}{12} = \frac{2}{24}$$

3. **Subtract the numerators.** Once the fractions are converted, the subtraction is similar to the addition. *Subtract only the numerators,* place them over the common denominator, and reduce if possible.

$$\frac{9}{24} - \frac{2}{24} = \frac{7}{24}$$

NOTE: When faced with mixed numbers, you can *either* subtract the whole numbers separately and then add them to the difference of the remaining fractions (and reduce) *or* convert the mixed numbers to an improper fraction and subtract the fractions as above.

EXERCISE 1.3 SUBTRACTION OF FRACTIONS

(Answers may be found in Appendix B.)

Directions: Subtract the following fractions and reduce if possible.

1. $\frac{3}{4} - \frac{1}{4} =$

2. $\frac{1}{8} - \frac{1}{12} =$

3. $\frac{1}{12} - \frac{1}{16} =$

4. $6\frac{2}{3} - 5\frac{3}{4} =$

5. $8\frac{1}{12} - 3\frac{1}{4} =$

6. $10\frac{1}{2} - 5\frac{3}{4} =$

7. $2\frac{1}{8} - \frac{5}{12} =$

8. $7\frac{1}{5} - 4\frac{1}{2} =$

9. $100\frac{1}{33} - 33\frac{1}{3} =$

10. $250\frac{1}{20} - 175\frac{1}{25} =$

1.4 MULTIPLICATION OF FRACTIONS

Multiplying fractions is quite simple. Fractions can be multiplied without converting to a common denominator. There are only two major steps to multiply fractions. Look at the following example:

$$\frac{2}{4} \times \frac{1}{3} = ?$$

1. Simply multiply the numerators together and then the denominators together.

$$\frac{2 \times 1}{4 \times 3} = \frac{2}{12}$$

2. Reduce if possible.

$$\frac{2}{12} \div \frac{2}{2} = \frac{1}{6}$$

Fractions can also be multiplied by whole numbers. To perform this computation, convert the whole number to a fraction and multiply as shown. Remember to reduce if possible.

$$\frac{1}{8} \times 2 = ?$$

Convert 2 to a fraction, multiply, and reduce.

$$\frac{1}{8} \times \frac{2}{1} = \frac{2}{8} \qquad \frac{2}{8} \div \frac{2}{2} = \frac{1}{4}$$

NOTE: Mixed numbers are different with multiplication. You must convert mixed numbers to an improper fraction and multiply the fractions as above. Of course, reduce all answers to their lowest terms.

EXERCISE 1.4 MULTIPLICATION OF FRACTIONS

(Answers may be found in Appendix B.)

Directions: Multiply the following fractions and reduce if possible.

1. $\frac{2}{4} \times \frac{1}{2} =$

2. $\frac{1}{2} \times \frac{1}{3} =$

3. $\frac{1}{8} \times \frac{1}{12} =$

4. $\frac{1}{2} \times \frac{1}{4} =$

5. $1\frac{1}{2} \times 2\frac{1}{4} =$

6. $3\frac{1}{3} \times \frac{1}{3} =$

7. $2\frac{2}{3} \times 4\frac{1}{2} =$

8. $5\frac{1}{6} \times \frac{1}{8} =$

9. $\frac{1}{2} \times \frac{1}{3} \times \frac{1}{4} =$

10. $\frac{3}{4} \times \frac{5}{6} \times \frac{1}{12} =$

11. $\frac{5}{30} \times 12 =$

12. $\frac{5}{1} \times 81 =$

13. $\frac{250}{400} \times \frac{400}{10} \times \frac{60}{1} =$

14. $\frac{250}{1000} \times \frac{2}{1} \times \frac{60}{1} =$

15. $\frac{500}{2000} \times \frac{4}{1} \times 60 =$

16. $\frac{1000}{4000} \times 4 \times \frac{60}{1} =$

17. $\frac{100}{60} \times 15 =$

18. $\frac{200}{60} \times 60 =$

19. $\frac{250}{1000} \times \frac{4}{1} \times \frac{60}{1} =$

20. $\frac{25}{10} \times \frac{2}{1} \times \frac{6}{1} =$

1.5 DIVISION OF FRACTIONS

Division of common fractions requires familiarization with the terms dividend and divisor. Consider the following example:

$$\frac{3}{5} \div \frac{1}{3} = ?$$

The fraction $\frac{3}{5}$ is the **dividend,** the number to be divided, and $\frac{1}{3}$ is the **divisor.** There is a two-step method for dividing common fractions.

1. First, invert the divisor.

$$\frac{3}{5} \div \frac{3}{1} = ?$$

2. Next, change the problem to a multiplication problem and multiply. Reduce as necessary.

$$\frac{3}{5} \times \frac{3}{1} = \frac{9}{5}$$

$$\frac{9}{5} = 1\frac{4}{5}$$

Sometimes, the divisor may be a whole number. The whole number can be converted to a fraction, inverted, and then multiplied:

$$\frac{2}{3} \div 2 = ?$$

$$\frac{2}{3} \div \frac{2}{1} = ?$$

$$\frac{2}{3} \times \frac{1}{2} = \frac{2}{6}$$

$$\frac{2}{6} = \frac{1}{3}$$

EXERCISE 1.5 DIVISION OF FRACTIONS

(Answers may be found in Appendix B.)

Directions: Divide the following fractions and reduce if possible.

1. $\frac{1}{4} \div \frac{1}{2} =$

2. $\frac{1}{6} \div \frac{1}{3} =$

3. $\frac{1}{150} \div 2 =$

4. $\frac{1}{100} \div \frac{2}{3} =$

5. $\frac{1}{60} \div \frac{1}{2} =$

6. $\frac{1}{20} \div \frac{1}{3} =$

7. $\dfrac{1}{200} \div \dfrac{1}{2} =$

9. $10\dfrac{1}{2} \div 3 =$

8. $2\dfrac{1}{2} \div \dfrac{3}{4} =$

10. $150\dfrac{3}{4} \div \dfrac{1}{8} =$

CHAPTER 1 TEST: COMMON FRACTIONS

Fill in the blank.

1. A _____ is a mathematical representation for parts of a whole.

2. In a common fraction, the bottom number, or the _____, represents the total number of equal parts in the whole.

3. The top number, or the _____, represents the number of parts being considered.

4. In a(n) _____ fraction, the numerator is **smaller** than the denominator.

5. In a(n) _____ fraction, the numerator is **larger** than the denominator.

6. Any number over itself in a common fraction equals _____.

7. Any whole number can be expressed as a fraction by placing it as a numerator over the denominator of _____.

8. _____ numbers are divisible only by themselves and the number 1.

When adding or subtracting common fractions, fractions must be converted to the 9. _____ 10. _____ denominator.

Solve the following.

11. $\dfrac{1}{5} + \dfrac{2}{10} =$

16. $\dfrac{500}{1000} \times 4 \times 60 =$

12. $\dfrac{3}{8} + \dfrac{1}{9} =$

17. $\dfrac{300}{100} \times \dfrac{60}{1} =$

13. $\dfrac{3}{4} - \dfrac{2}{8} =$

18. $\dfrac{1}{20} \div \dfrac{1}{3} =$

14. $\dfrac{7}{10} - \dfrac{2}{5} =$

19. $\dfrac{1}{150} \div 2 =$

15. $\dfrac{250}{400} \times \dfrac{400}{10} \times \dfrac{60}{1} =$

20. $\dfrac{1}{60} \div \dfrac{1}{2} =$

Decimal Fractions

OBJECTIVES

In order to work dosage calculation problems as an emergency health care provider, you should be able to:

1. Define a decimal fraction.

2. List and identify the decimal places.

3. Define and identify a decimal point.

4. Demonstrate the use of a zero as a place holder.

5. Round off a decimal fraction to an identified place.

6. Add decimal fractions.

7. Subtract decimal fractions.

8. Multiply decimal fractions.

9. Divide decimal fractions.

INTRODUCTION

- *How is a decimal fraction different from a common fraction?*
- *How do you round off a decimal fraction?*
- *Do the decimal points have to be lined up when multiplying?*

These are questions that anyone could be asking about decimal fractions. In this chapter, these questions and many others will be addressed as we review decimal fractions. There are plenty of practice problems with answers in the back of the book.

Even while they teach, men learn.
—Seneca—

2.1 DECIMAL FRACTION FUNDAMENTALS

Decimal fractions are another way to express parts of a whole. They are fractions based upon the power of 10 or multiples of 10, such as 10, 100, 1000. The root *deci-* originates with the Latin *decimus,* which means "tenth." A **decimal point** separates the whole number from the decimal fraction. To the left of the decimal point are the whole number places, and to the right are the fractional places. Each place to the right and to the left of the decimal point has a name. The fractional places represent a fraction whose denominator is a power of 10 (see Figure 2.1). The number 1234.5678 is shown in the figure. The 5 in the tenths place could also be expressed as $\frac{5}{10}$ or the 6 in the hundredths place as $\frac{6}{100}$ and so on. The entire number could also be expressed as:

$$1234\frac{5678}{10000}$$

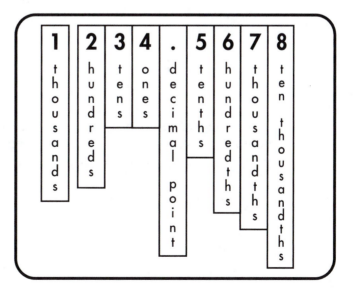

Figure 2.1 Decimal places.

The Decimal Point

When stating decimal numbers, use the word *point* for the decimal point. The number 2.5 would be stated, "two point five." When discussing money, the decimal point is stated using the word *and*. The dollar amount $2.50 is stated, "two dollars and fifty cents." When performing mathematical problems with decimal numbers, zeros that are to the right of the decimal point that are not between other numbers can be eliminated. In the number 2.50, the zero can be eliminated. It has no value. However, in the number 2.05, the zero gives value to the number and cannot be eliminated.

Another very important feature of the decimal is quite important to the health care professional. When dealing with decimal fractions that do not have an associated whole number, a zero must always be documented and stated before the decimal. For example, when expressing the decimal fraction five-tenths, it is documented 0.5 and is stated, "zero point five." This draws attention to the very important decimal point and helps to eliminate errors in drug dosage administration.

Rounding Off

Most syringes and other measuring devices used in emergency and prehospital care measure accurately to a tenth or, at most, to a hundredth. Because of this, the emergency care provider frequently needs to *round off* decimal fractions. Rounding off is the process of converting a long decimal fraction to a more practical one with fewer decimal places.

To round off a decimal fraction, identify the place to which the number is to be rounded. If the number in the place immediately to the right is 5 or greater, then add one to the place in question. Then, drop the numbers following the place in question. For example, the number 1.246 is to be rounded to the hundredth.

Identify the place to be rounded:

1.2**4**6

Is the number to the right five or greater?

1.2**46**

If so, add one to the place in question and drop the following numbers:

1.25

If the number to the right of the place in question is less than 5, then the number in question stays the same. The number 6.4299 needs to be rounded to the nearest tenth. First, identify the place to be rounded:

6.**4**299

Is the number to the right less than 5?

6.4**2**99

If so, drop the numbers to the right of the place to be rounded:

6.4

EXERCISE 2.1 DECIMAL FRACTION FUNDAMENTALS

(Answers may be found in Appendix B.)

In the following decimal fractions, identify the place that is bolded:

1. 298.32**5**

2. **1**345.25

3. **0**.5

4. 20.651**9**

5. 0.5**5**

6. 5.**5**

7. **1**2.1

8. 40.7**6**32

9. 75.3**3**3

10. 5**0**.05

Round the following decimal fractions to the nearest *hundredth:*

11. 25.333

12. 36.006

13. 50.348

14. 1723.401989

15. 0.009

Round the following decimal fractions to the nearest *tenth:*

16. 25.433

17. 100.549

18. 75.19

19. 9.999

20. 10.01

2.2 ADDITION OF DECIMAL FRACTIONS

When we deposit our paycheck into a checking account, we are adding decimal fractions. The key to adding decimal fractions is lining up the decimals vertically. For example, the numbers 1.25, 3.5, and 0.33 need to be added together. Use this simple three-step method:

1. Line up the decimal fractions on the decimal.

$$
\begin{array}{r}
1.25 \\
3.5 \\
+\ 0.33 \\
\hline
\end{array}
$$

2. Add place holders (if needed) and add. Some people like to add zeros at the end of decimal fractions as place holders before adding. This helps to

eliminate mistakes. When this is done, add the numbers vertically, carry-ing over as needed. The decimal carries straight down vertically.

$$
\begin{array}{r}
1.25 \\
3.50 \quad \leftarrow \text{zero place holder added} \\
+ \ 0.33 \\
\hline
5.08
\end{array}
$$

3. Now that you have the answer, you could round the sum to the place that your text or dosage calculation requires.

EXERCISE 2.2 ADDITION OF DECIMAL FRACTIONS

(Answers may be found in Appendix B.)

Directions: Add the following decimal fractions. Round to the nearest hundredth.

1. $2.5 + 4.6 + 20.9 =$

2. $10.2 + 32.3 + 1.45 =$

3. $6.95 + 7.5 + 12.125 =$

4. $0.01 + 0.25 + 2.496 =$

5. $1.25 + 0.50 + 72.28 =$

6. $10.2 + 0.02 + 3 =$

7. $16 + 2.75 + 7.005 + 0.084 =$

8. $0.0001 + 1.05 + 4.006 + 2 =$

9. $5.0 + 2.1 + 0.01 + 0.45 + 2.56 =$

10. $1.5 + 0.25 + 3.6 + 2.45 + 1.75 =$

2.3 SUBTRACTION OF DECIMAL FRACTIONS

When we write a check or use an automatic teller machine, we are sub-tracting decimals from our account. Subtracting decimal fractions employs the same rules as addition. Align numbers in a vertical column along the decimal point. Add place holders to avoid mistakes. Look at the following example:

$$4.10 \quad \leftarrow \text{zero place holder added}$$
$$\underline{- \ 0.48}$$
$$3.62$$

EXERCISE 2.3 SUBTRACTION OF DECIMAL FRACTIONS

(Answers may be found in Appendix B.)

Directions: Subtract the following decimal fractions. Round to the nearest hundredth.

1. $1000 - 250.5 =$ 6. $0.5 - 0.25 =$ 11. $1 - 0.1 =$

2. $10.2 - 3.1 =$ 7. $33.3 - 0.5 =$ 12. $1 - 0.5 =$

3. $100 - 97.26 =$ 8. $16.3 - 12.5 =$ 13. $1 - 0.7 =$

4. $1.25 - 0.34 =$ 9. $2.5 - 0.95 =$ 14. $5 - 2.5 =$

5. $500 - 125.75 =$ 10. $4.92 - 1.64 =$ 15. $3 - 1.5 =$

2.4 MULTIPLICATION OF DECIMAL FRACTIONS

When multiplying decimal fractions, it is not necessary to align decimal points. Simply write and multiply the problem like any other multiplication problem. Leave the decimal points in their original places. The question is usually where to place the decimal point in the product (answer). Let's see how the problem 4.5×2.25 would be calculated:

1. Write the problem like any other multiplication problem.

2. Multiply the numbers like any other multiplication problem.

3. Add the number of decimal places in the numbers being multiplied. Start from the right of the product and move that number of places to the left. This is where the decimal place belongs.

$$
\begin{array}{r}
4.5 \quad \leftarrow \text{1 decimal place} \\
\underline{\times \ 2.25} \quad \leftarrow \text{2 decimal places} \\
225 \\
900 \\
\underline{+ \ 9000} \\
10.125 \quad \leftarrow \text{3 decimal places in product}
\end{array}
$$

You may now round the product to the place that your text or dosage calculation requires.

EXERCISE 2.4 MULTIPLICATION OF DECIMAL FRACTIONS

(Answers may be found in Appendix B.)

Directions: Multiply the following decimal fractions. Round to the nearest hundredth.

1. $1.5 \times 2 =$	6. $0.0345 \times 4.6 =$	11. $100 \times 0.45 =$
2. $0.25 \times 1.25 =$	7. $9.26 \times 7 =$	12. $200 \times 0.45 =$
3. $0.75 \times 4 =$	8. $31.286 \times 8.01 =$	13. $100 \times 1.5 =$
4. $5.85 \times 2 =$	9. $0.0033 \times 9.02 =$	14. $100 \times 0.1 =$
5. $0.625 \times 3.3 =$	10. $16.325 \times 0.006 =$	15. $100 \times 0.01 =$

2.5 DIVISION OF DECIMAL FRACTIONS

When dividing decimal fractions, it is first necessary to determine where the decimal place will be in the quotient (answer). This depends on where the decimal point is in the dividend (the number being divided) *and* whether the divisor (the number that divides) is either a whole number or a decimal fraction.

When the divisor is a whole number, the decimal place for the quotient belongs directly over the decimal place of the dividend. The problem $8.54 \div 2$ needs to be solved. Place the decimal point in the quotient directly above the dividend's decimal point, as shown:

$$\text{divisor} \rightarrow 2\overline{)8.54} \quad \begin{array}{l} 4.27 \quad \leftarrow \text{quotient} \\ \phantom{2\overline{)8.54}} \leftarrow \text{dividend} \end{array}$$

Sometimes the divisor is a decimal fraction. When this is the case, the divisor must be converted to a whole number to work the problem. For example, the problem $28.35 \div 2.5$ must be solved. For the divisor 2.5 to be converted to a whole number, it must be multiplied by 10. Whenever the divisor in the problem is multiplied by a number, the dividend must also be multiplied by that number. The 2.5 becomes 25, and the 28.35 becomes 283.5.

An easier way to remember how to do this requires no math at all. Simply move the decimal point in the divisor as many places to the right that will change it to a whole number. Then, move the decimal point in the dividend the same number of places to the right, adding zeros when necessary. Look at the following problem:

$$\text{divisor} \rightarrow 2.5\overline{)28.35}$$

becomes

$$\begin{array}{r} 11.34 \quad \leftarrow \text{quotient} \\ 25\overline{)283.50} \quad \leftarrow \text{dividend} \end{array}$$

NOTE: If a quotient does not divide out evenly, calculate to one place beyond the place you will round, then round off the answer.

EXERCISE 2.5 DIVISION OF DECIMAL FRACTIONS

(Answers may be found in Appendix B.)

Directions: Multiply the following decimal fractions. Round to the nearest hundredth.

1. $100 \div 3.5 =$

2. $15.5 \div 1.5 =$

3. $20.5 \div 2.4 =$

4. $56.5 \div 0.02 =$

5. $2.5 \div 0.001 =$

6. $33.3 \div 3.3 =$

7. $25.1 \div 5.02 =$

8. $500.75 \div 12.5 =$

9. $10.075 \div 4.5 =$

10. $0.065 \div 15 =$

CHAPTER 2 TEST: DECIMAL FRACTIONS

1. Decimal fractions separate whole numbers from fractions by means of a _____ _____.

2. In the number 1234.5678, the 5 is in the _____ place.

3. In the number 1234.5678, the 6 is in the _____ place.

4. When dealing with decimal fractions that do not have an associated whole number, a _____ must always be documented and stated before the decimal.

5. _____ _____ is the process of converting a long decimal fraction to a more practical one with fewer decimal places.

Round the following to the nearest tenth.

6. 50.549

7. 9.968

8. 10.01

Solve the following.

9. $20.002 + 0.02 + 2.2 =$ 15. $220 \times 0.45 =$

10. $0.125 + 0.75 + 0.025 =$ 16. $100 \times 0.45 =$

11. $0.25 + 0.25 =$ 17. $100 \times 0.01 =$

12. $1 - 0.1 =$ 18. $33.3 \div 3.3 =$

13. $5 - 2.5 =$ 19. $99 \div 0.45 =$

14. $1 - 0.5 =$ 20. $10 \div 0.5 =$

chapter 3

Ratios and Proportions

OBJECTIVES

In order to work dosage calculation problems as an emergency health care provider, you should be able to:

1. Define and identify a ratio.

2. Define and identify a proportion.

3. Define and identify the extremes in a proportion.

4. Define and identify the means in a proportion.

5. Solve for X in proportion problems.

6. Solve for X using cross-multiplication.

INTRODUCTION

- *What is a ratio?*
- *What is a proportion?*
- *How do ratios compare to common fractions?*
- *How is cross-multiplication similar to ratios and proportions?*

The answer to these questions and others will help you solve a majority of the dosage calculation problems you encounter in emergency care. Along with understanding ratios and proportions, you will learn how to solve for X and review the cross-multiplication technique. Pay careful attention to the information in this chapter and you will have a good foundation for the chapters ahead.

> *Never, never, never, never give up.*
> **—Sir Winston Churchill—**

3.1 RATIOS AND PROPORTIONS

So far we have discussed parts of a whole as common fractions and decimal fractions. Using ratios is another method for expressing parts of a whole. A **ratio** is a comparison of two numbers that are somehow related to one another. The numbers are separated by a colon (:), which is stated "is to." A vial of medication could have 20 milligrams of a drug in 10 milliliters. This can be expressed as the ratio

$$20 \text{ mg} : 10 \text{ mL}$$

This would be stated, "twenty milligrams is to ten milliliters." It can also be expressed as the fraction $\frac{20 \text{ mg}}{10 \text{ mL}}$ or, as is seen on medication vials, as 20 mg/10 mL. A ratio is simply a fractional number expressed in a slightly different fashion.

When two ratios are equal, they can be expressed as a proportion. A **proportion** consists of two related ratios separated by an equal sign (=) or a double colon (::), which means the two ratios are equal. The double colon is stated, "as." For example, we have a syringe of the medication listed above that has 10 milligrams of drug in 5 milliliters of volume. The comparison of the vial to the syringe can be expressed as the proportion

$$20 \text{ mg} : 10 \text{ mL} :: 10 \text{ mg} : 5 \text{ mL}$$

$$\text{(vial)} \qquad \text{(syringe)}$$

This would be stated, "twenty milligrams is to ten milliliters as ten milligrams is to five milliliters." It is essential that the ratios (units of mg/mL) are in the same sequence on both sides of the double colon for it to be a proportion. The numbers on the ends of the proportion (20, 5) are called the **extremes.** The numbers in the middle (10, 10) are called the **means.** In a proportion, the product of the extremes equals the product of the means. If we multiply the extremes, then multiply the means, the answers will be equal:

$$20 \times 5 = 100 \text{ (extremes)}$$

$$10 \times 10 = 100 \text{ (means)}$$

Since it is critical that the extremes and the means not be confused, it's helpful to use the following memory cue. The *means* are in the *middle* of a proportion. One definition of the word *mean* is the middle point. "Means" and "middle" both start with the letter "m." The *extremes* are the farthest *ends* of anything. Both these words start with the letter "e." This also emphasizes the importance of keeping the two ratios in proper order when describing them as a proportion. If the order of the two ratios is not the same, the equation will not be accurate or make any sense. In other words, the answer you get will be wrong. So, when performing dosage calculations, pay careful attention to the order of the ratios in a proportion.

EXERCISE 3.1 RATIOS AND PROPORTIONS

(Answers may be found in Appendix B.)

Directions: Solve the following ratio and proportion problems.

Express the following common fractions as ratios:

1. $\dfrac{1}{10}$

2. $\dfrac{4}{5}$

3. $\dfrac{200}{10}$

4. $\dfrac{100}{5}$

5. $\dfrac{500}{10}$

Express the following ratios as common fractions:

6. 1:2

7. 1:250

8. 8:5

9. 10:1

10. 3:1

In the following proportions, identify the extremes:

11. 1:2::5:10

12. 100:5::10:0.5

13. 40:10::20:5

14. 2:1::10:5

15. 10:1000::1:100

In the following proportions, identify the means:

16. 1:2::5:10

17. 100:5::10:0.5

18. 40:10::20:5

19. 2:1::10:5

20. 10:1000::1:100

3.2 PROPORTIONS AND CROSS-MULTIPLICATION

Understanding the principles of ratios and proportions can help solve for any one missing element of the proportion. This technique is used to solve many of the drug dosage calculations that will be found in prehospital/emergency care and testing. Look at the proportion discussed in Section 3.1:

$$20 \text{ mg} : 10 \text{ mL} :: 10 \text{ mg} : 5 \text{ mL}$$

$$\text{(vial)} \qquad \text{(syringe)}$$

Suppose we know how many milliliters are in the syringe, but we do not know how many milligrams are in that syringe. However, we do know the syringe was drawn from the vial. How can the number of milligrams be determined? Here is a simple three-step method:

1. Write the proportion with X as the unknown.

NOTE: Make sure the units are in the same sequence:

$$20 \text{ mg} : 10 \text{ mL} :: X \text{ mg} : 5 \text{ mL}$$

2. Multiply the means. Multiply the extremes. In algebraic equations X is usually put on the left side:

$$10 X = 20 \times 5$$

$$10 X = 100$$

3. In order to solve for X, divide both sides by the number to be multiplied by X; in this case, the number 10:

$$\frac{10X}{10} = \frac{100}{10}$$

$$X = \textbf{10 mg}$$

Cross-Multiplication

Some people prefer working with common fractions. Recall that proportions can easily be converted to common fractions. The proportion example above can also be expressed as two common fractions that are equal to each other:

$$\frac{20 \text{ mg}}{10 \text{ mL}} = \frac{10 \text{ mg}}{5 \text{ mL}}$$

Solving proportion problems is similar to a process most of us learned in elementary school known as cross-multiplication (see the discussion of cross-multiplication on p. 13). If you prefer to work with common fractions, this method may have greater appeal, though mathematically it is the same equation. Cross-multiplication or cross products is a technique used to solve for any one unknown part of two equal common fractions. When two common fractions are equal, multiplying the denominator of a fraction on the left side of the equal sign by the numerator of the fraction on the right side equals multiplying the numerator of the one on the left by the denominator of the one on the right. This application was used in Chapter 1 to prove that two common fractions were equal to each other. Now, that same technique can be used to solve for X. Look at the following example:

$$\frac{20 \text{ mg}}{10 \text{ mL}} = \frac{X \text{ mg}}{5 \text{ mL}}$$

1. To solve for X using cross-multiplication, multiply the denominator on the left (10 mL) by the numerator on the right (X mg):

$$10X =$$

2. Now, multiply the numerator on the left (20 mg) by the denominator on the right (5 mL). Solve for X:

$$10X = 20 \times 5$$
$$10X = 100$$
$$\frac{10X}{10} = \frac{100}{10}$$
$$X = \textbf{10 mg}$$

The basic algebraic equation is still the same as that used in the proportion equation. Some people just "see" a problem one way and not the other. Use whichever method you prefer. *How* you get an answer is not usually tested. Getting the answer *right* is!

EXERCISE 3.2 PROPORTIONS AND CROSS-MULTIPLICATION

(Answers may be found in Appendix B.)

Directions: Solve for X in the following proportion problems.

1. $5:10::X:2$

2. $3:6::6:X$

3. $40:X::80:10$

4. $\dfrac{5}{200} = \dfrac{X}{4000}$

5. $5:15::6:X$

6. $X:5000::10:500$

7. $60:2::30:X$

8. $50:1::150:X$

9. $6:2::12:X$

10. $\dfrac{1000}{250} = \dfrac{X}{1}$

11. $100:10::10:X$

12. $10:1::50:X$

13. $0.75:X::1:1$

14. $\dfrac{X}{5} = \dfrac{15}{1}$

15. $1:10::0.5:X$

16. $\dfrac{60}{2} = \dfrac{30}{X}$

17. $1:X::0.1:1$

18. $\dfrac{200}{250} = \dfrac{X}{1}$

19. $150:3::300:X$

20. $X:2::1:0.4$

1. A _____ is a comparison of two numbers that are somehow related to one another.

2. The numbers in a ratio are separated by a _____.

3. A _____ consists of two equal ratios.

4. The two ratios in a proportion are separated by a _____ _____.

5. The numbers on the two ends of a proportion are called the _____.

Solve the following.

6. $5:10::X:2$

7. $60:2::30:X$

8. $150:1::300:X$

9. $1000:250::X:1$

10. $200:250::X:1$

chapter 4

Percentages

In order to work dosage calculation problems as an emergency health care provider, you should be able to:

1. Define and identify a percent.

2. Define and identify a weight/weight percent.

3. Define and identify a volume/volume percent.

4. Define and identify a weight/volume percent.

5. Define and identify a ratio solution.

6. Find the percent of a number.

7. Find the percent one number is of another.

8. Find the total number that another known number is the percent of.

INTRODUCTION

- *What is a solution?*
- *Can a solution be accurately defined as concentrated or dilute?*

- *What is a weight/volume percent?*
- *What is a ratio solution?*
- *Just what does **percent** mean, anyway?*

Prehospital and emergency personnel work with solutions and percentages every day. Bags of I.V. fluid, drugs, tablets, and even oxygen—all these are examples of solutions that could have varying concentrations. In this chapter, we will explore the language of solutions, how concentrations are expressed, and work some simple percent problems.

> *To avoid all mistakes in the conduct of great enterprises*
> *is beyond man's powers.*
> **—Fabius Maximus—**

4.1 PERCENTAGE FUNDAMENTALS

Percent

So far we have discussed the parts of a whole as fractions, decimal fractions, ratios, and proportions. An alternative method for expressing parts of a whole is **percentage,** which is derived from the Latin *per centum* meaning "by the hundred." Percentage indicates the weight or volume of solute present in 100 units of solution. Percents (or per cents) are merely fractions with denominators of 100. They are expressed with a percent sign (%), which means "for every hundred." For instance, "5%" means 5 for every 100 parts. It may also be written as $\frac{5}{100}$ or 5:100 or 0.05. The symbol can be used with a whole number (1%), a common fraction $\left(\frac{1}{4}\%\right)$, a mixed number $\left(10\frac{1}{2}\%\right)$, or a decimal fraction (0.9%).

NOTE: There need not actually be 100 total units for a number or solution to be expressed as a percentage.

There are three ways in which percentage concentration may be expressed:

1. **Weight/weight percent** expresses the number of grams of solute in 100 grams of solution. This means that the *total* weight of both components equals 100 grams.

2. **Volume/volume percent** expresses the number of milliliters of solute in a total volume of 100 mL of solution.

3. **Weight/volume percent** is the most commonly used percentage concentration with emergency medications. It expresses the number of grams of solute in a total volume of 100 mL of solution. When concentration is expressed as a percentage, it is assumed to be weight/volume unless otherwise indicated.

For example, 50% dextrose is a common emergency drug expressed as a weight/volume percentage (see Figure 4.1). This means that there are

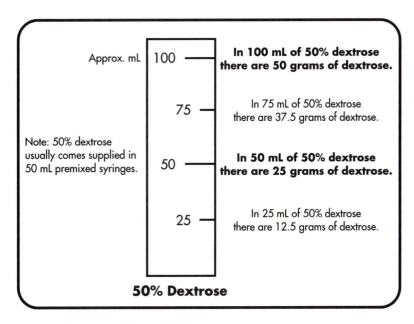

Figure 4.1 Weight/volume percent.

50 grams (50 g) of dextrose in every 100 milliliters (100 mL) of the solution. For more discussion about solutions, see Chapter 12, Solutions and Dilutions.

Ratio Solutions

Another way to express concentration in a solution is by using a ratio. These are not as common as weight/volume percent, but there are still a number of medications on ambulances and in emergency centers that use ratios to express concentration. **Ratio solutions** are expressed as 1 gram of a drug in 100 mL, 1000 mL, or 10 000 mL of solvent. Epinephrine is a common drug expressed as a ratio solution. This drug is commonly supplied as 1:1000 and 1:10 000 epinephrine. This is how the ratios will appear and what they mean:

$$1:1000 = 1 \text{ g per } 1000 \text{ mL}$$

$$1:10\,000 = 1 \text{ g per } 10\,000 \text{ mL}$$

Look at the ratio solutions expressed as fractions:

$$\mathbf{1:1000} = \frac{1 \text{ g}}{1000 \text{ mL}} = \frac{1000 \text{ mg}}{1000 \text{ mL}} = \frac{1 \text{ mg}}{1 \text{ mL}}$$

The 1 milligram per 1 milliliter concentration is the origin of the medical jargon of "one to one epi." Remember that for proper documentation, the correct ratio solution expression should be 1:1000 or the proper weight/volume percentage of $\frac{1 \text{ mg}}{1 \text{ mL}}$ should be used.

$$\mathbf{1:10\,000} = \frac{1 \text{ g}}{10\,000 \text{ mL}} = \frac{1000 \text{ mg}}{10\,000 \text{ mL}} = \frac{1 \text{ mg}}{10 \text{ mL}}$$

The 1 milligram per 10 milliliter concentration is the origin of the medical jargon of "one to ten epi." Remember that for proper documentation, the correct ratio solution expression should be 1 : 10 000 or the proper weight/volume percentage of $\frac{1\,mg}{10\,mL}$ should be used.

EXERCISE 4.1 PERCENTAGE FUNDAMENTALS

(Answers may be found in Appendix B.)

Directions: Answer the following questions about percentage and ratio solutions.

1. The percent sign (%) means:

    a. "for every hundred"
    b. "for every thousand"
    c. "divided by one hundred thousand"
    d. none of the above

2. Percents are merely fractions with denominators of:

    a. 10
    b. 100
    c. 1000
    d. none of the above

3. The percent that expresses the number of grams of solute in a total volume of 100 mL of solution is a:

    a. weight/weight percent
    b. volume/volume percent
    c. weight/volume percent
    d. any of the above

4. A medication label reads, "2% Lidocaine." This means there are 2 _____ of Lidocaine in every _____ mL of solution.

    a. grams/100
    b. milligrams/100
    c. micrograms/10
    d. none of the above

5. "5%" means:

    a. 5 for every 100 parts
    b. 50 for every 100 parts
    c. 5 for every 1000 parts
    d. 50 for every 1000 parts

6. A ratio solution expresses 1 gram of a drug in 100 mL, 1000 mL, or 10 000 mL of solvent.

    a. True
    b. False

4.2 PERCENT PROBLEMS

The following three basic percent problems help prepare us for percent problems involving drug dosage calculations and may help you solve questions about exams. The first type will seek the percent of a number, the second is looking for the percent one number is of another, and the third type is looking to find the number that another number is the percent of. This may seem confusing at first, so we address each one individually.

1. **Find the percent of a number.** This type of percent problem can be compared to a test that would be taken by a student. The test will have 200 questions, and 70% is passing. How many questions must the student get *right* to achieve a 70% grade? To solve this problem, the percentage must be converted to a decimal fraction and the word "of" changed to "multiply."

Example: What is 70% of 200?

    a. Convert 70% to a decimal fraction (see Chapter 5, Putting It All Together, p. 44):

$$70\% = 0.7$$

    b. Substitute "of" with "multiply" and solve:

$$0.7 \times 200 = \mathbf{140}$$

2. **Find the percent one number is of another.** In this type of percent problem, the word "of" will mean "divide." It is a twist on the first type of percent problem. It could be compared to our test from above. In this instance, the number of questions the student answered correctly is known and the number of questions on the test are known. The question is what percent grade did the student achieve? The answer will be a decimal fraction that needs to be converted to a percent.

Example: 140 is what percent of 200?

    a. Substitute "is what percent of" with "divided by" and solve:

$$\begin{array}{r} 0.7 \\ 200\overline{)140.0} \end{array}$$

    b. Convert the decimal fraction answer to a percent:

$$0.7 = 70\%$$

The same question could also be worded: "What percent of 200 is 140?" It would be solved exactly like the previous example. It is the same question worded a little differently.

3. **Find the number that another number is the percent of.** In this type of percent problem, the percent will need to be changed to a decimal fraction and divided into the number. Using our example of the test, the percent grade is known, and the number of questions answered correctly is known. How many questions that are on the test needs to be determined.

Example: 70% of what number is 140?

    a.   Convert 70% to a decimal fraction:

$$70\% = 0.7$$

    b.   Divide the remaining number by the decimal fraction:

$$0.7\overline{)140} = 70\overline{)14000} \quad (200)$$

EXERCISE 4.2 PERCENTAGE FUNDAMENTALS

(Answers may be found in Appendix B.)

Directions: Solve the following percent problems.

1.   What is 5% of 250?

2.   25 is what percent of 500?

3.   50% of what number is 25?

4.   What is 80% of 150?

5.   12.5 is what percent of 250?

6.   15% of what number is 12?

7.   What is 90% of 225?

8.   120 is what percent of 150?

9.   75% of what number is 150?

10.   What percent of 500 is 25?

Putting It All Together: Fraction Conversions

In order to work dosage calculation problems as an emergency health care provider, you should be able to:

1. Convert common fractions to decimal fractions.

2. Convert decimal fractions to common fractions.

3. Convert decimal fractions to percentages.

4. Convert percentages to decimal fractions.

5. Convert a common fraction to a percentage.

6. Convert percentages to common fractions.

7. Convert a ratio to a common fraction.

INTRODUCTION

- *How are common fractions converted to decimals?*
- *How are percentages converted to common fractions?*
- *How can a ratio be converted to any other fraction?*

All drug dosage calculations will involve parts of wholes. You must be able to convert between the different types of fractions. In this chapter, the conversions between fractions will be discussed. There is a fraction conversion table at the end of the chapter that can be used for practice.

> *Where there is much desire to learn, there of necessity*
> *will be much arguing, much writing, many opinions; for*
> *opinion in good men is but knowledge in the making.*
> **—John Milton—**

5.1 FRACTION CONVERSIONS

Drug dosage calculations in emergency care deal with parts of a whole, concentrations, and solutions. To accurately determine answers to these problems, it will be necessary to convert between fractions. When a dosage is a common fraction and a decimal fraction is needed, how will it be converted? Or if an answer is in percent and needs to be a ratio, how will it be converted? The following seven conversions are the most common types of conversions that the emergency care provider will need to be able to perform.

1. **Converting common fractions to decimal fractions.** When calculating drug dosages, it may be necessary to convert common fractions into decimal fractions in order to administer a drug. This is achieved by dividing the numerator by the denominator and adding zeros as needed. What if a drug dosage calculation ended with the answer $\frac{1}{2}$ and the syringe to be used was measuring in decimals?

   Divide the numerator by the denominator:

   $$\frac{1}{2} = 1 \div 2 = \mathbf{0.5}$$

   Mixed numbers may also be encountered that need to be converted to decimals. Simply convert the fraction part of the mixed number to a decimal fraction and add it to the whole number. For example, the mixed number $40\frac{3}{4}$ is the answer to a drug dosage calculation. The syringe to be used measures in decimal fractions. Convert the $\frac{3}{4}$ to the decimal 0.75, and add it to the 40 for an answer of 40.75.

2. **Converting decimal fractions to common fractions.** This process can be reversed. The number 30.25 needs to be converted to a mixed number. The decimal fraction part of the number can be converted to the common fraction $\frac{25}{100}$ and then reduced to $\frac{1}{4}$. The converted number is now $30\frac{1}{4}$. It could also be converted to the improper fraction of $\frac{121}{4}$ if needed.

3. **Converting decimal fractions to percentages.** A drug dosage calculation ends with a decimal fraction and a percent is needed. How can this be converted? To convert a decimal fraction to a percent, multiply the decimal fraction by 100 and add a percent sign.

Example: Convert 0.44 to a percentage.

$$0.44 \times 100 = \textbf{44\%}$$

NOTE: Remember to add the percent sign.

There is an easier conversion technique. Simply move the decimal point two places to the *right* and add a percent sign.

Example: Convert 0.125 to a percentage.

Move the decimal point two places to the right and add a percent sign:

12.5%

4. **Converting percentages to decimal fractions.** To change a percentage to a decimal fraction, multiply by 0.01 and remove the percent sign.

Example: Convert 85% to a decimal fraction.

$$85\% \times 0.01 = \textbf{0.85}$$

Of course, the simpler technique from above can be reversed. Now, simply move the decimal point two places to the *left* and drop the percent sign.

Example: Convert 66.7% to a decimal fraction.

Move the decimal point two places to the left and drop the percent sign:

0.667

5. **Converting a common fraction to a percentage.** A drug dosage calculation using the cross-multiplication technique ends with a fraction. What if a percentage is requested? The process of converting a common fraction to a percent takes two steps. First, the fraction is converted to a decimal (see conversion 1 above). Then, the decimal is converted to a percentage as in conversion 3 above. Remember to add the percent sign and round to the appropriate place.

Example: Convert $\frac{1}{3}$ to a percentage.

    a.   Convert $\frac{1}{3}$ to a decimal fraction (see conversion 1):

$$\frac{1}{3} = 0.33$$

    b.   Convert 0.33 to a percentage (see conversion 3):

$$0.33 = \textbf{33\%}$$

6. **Converting percentages to common fractions.** If an answer to a percent problem needs to be expressed as a common fraction, reverse the process and then add the step of reducing the fraction.

Example: Convert 50% to a common fraction.

a. Convert 50% to a decimal fraction (see conversion 3):

$$50\% = 0.5$$

b. Convert 0.5 to a common fraction (see conversion 2):

$$\frac{50}{100}$$

c. Reduce the fraction:

$$\frac{50}{100} = \frac{1}{2}$$

7. **Ratios.** Remember a ratio is just another way to express a common fraction. The first number in a ratio is the numerator and the second number is the denominator. The ratio $3:1$ is the common fraction $\frac{3}{1}$. If conversions from ratios are necessary, first convert the ratio to a common fraction and then follow the steps provided. If conversions to ratios are needed, convert to a reduced common fraction and then to a ratio.

EXERCISE 5.1 FRACTION CONVERSIONS

(Answers may be found in Appendix B.)

Directions: Complete the following conversion chart.

Percentage	Decimal	Fraction	Ratio
1%			
	0.03		
		1/20	
			1 : 10
12.5%			
	0.25		
		1/3	
			3 : 4
100%			
	0.025		
		1/800	

SECTION TWO

SYSTEMS OF MEASUREMENT

This section reviews the systems of measurement that will most likely be encountered by the emergency care provider: the U.S. Customary Weights and Measures System and the metric system. A firm understanding of these systems is essential to accurate emergency dosage calculations.

If the comparison must be made,
if the distinction must be taken,
men are everything,
measures comparatively nothing.

—George Canning—

Systems of Measurement: An Historical Perspective

OBJECTIVES

In order to work dosage calculation problems and better understand the current status of systems of measurement in the United States, the emergency health care provider should be able to:

1. Name which branch of government has the power to set the standard for weights and measures in the United States.

2. Name and differentiate between the two systems of measurement used in the United States.

3. Define a unit.

4. Define a standard.

5. Identify and/or list examples of early systems of measurement.

6. Define "customary."

7. Identify and/or list examples of Roman contributions to modern systems of measurement.

8. Name the founder and father of the metric system.

9. Name the country where the metric system originated.

10. Chart the history of the metric system.

11. Identify the metric system by both its French and English names.

12. Define metric.

13. Chart the history of systems of measurement in the United States.

14. Define metrication.

15. Identify and recognize the Omnibus Trade and Competitiveness Act of 1988.

16. Identify and recognize Executive Order 12770, "Metric Usage in Federal Government Programs."

INTRODUCTION

- *How did systems of measurement develop?*
- *What was the reason for developing the metric system?*
- *Why does the United States have two systems of measurement?*

Dealing with two systems of measurement can be frustrating. By discovering the history of these systems, you can gain a better understanding of the current status of systems of measurement in the United States.

Man is the measure of all things.
—Protagoras—

6.1 AN HISTORICAL PERSPECTIVE

Article I, Section 8, of the U.S. Constitution gives Congress the power to set the standard for weights and measures in the United States. It says, "The Congress shall have power . . . to coin money, regulate the value thereof, and of foreign coin, and fix the standard of weights and measures . . . " Even though Congress has this power, it has been slow to establish a complete system. There are two systems of measurement used in the United States. An enduring, yet outmoded system, the **U.S. Customary Weights and Measures,** is still used in domestic and some commercial affairs. The other system, the **metric system,** is the primary system used in the sciences, medicine, most other countries, and for the most part, by the federal government. Many people become frustrated when solving problems with two systems of measurement. Why do we have to contend with two systems of measurement and the conversions

TABLE 6.1 The History of the Metric System Chart

1670	Gabriel Mouton forms the basics of the metric system.
1786	U.S. Congress establishes a decimal system of coinage.
1787	U.S. Constitution is ratified.
1790	Charles Maurice de Talleyrand-Perigord introduces a metric system plan to the National Assembly of France.
1790	The plan is delegated to the French Academy of Sciences and it establishes a decimal metric system.
1791	The French Academy of Sciences defines the unit of length to be called the *metre*.
1792	U. S. Congress passes Jefferson's Mint Act.
1795	France officially adopts the metric system.
1799	The French finalize definitions, and standards are created. Twelve nations attend diplomatic ceremonies. The United States is not one of them.
1805	Ferdinand Rudolf Hassler immigrates to the United States with his copy of the French standard of the meter.
1812	Napoleon decrees customary units legal again in France and suspends compulsory provisions of the metric system.
1814	The Troughton standard of the British yard is brought to the United States.
1840	The metric system is made mandatory in France.
1855	Copies of the British yard and the avoirdupois pound are presented to the United States.
1863	U. S. Congress establishes the National Academy of Sciences. Scientists begin pushing for legalization of the metric system.
1866	The president signs a bill legalizing the metric system in the United States.
1875	The Diplomatic Conference on the Meter (the Convention of the Meter) is held in Paris. The United States participates and the Treaty of the Metre is signed.
1878	The Convention of the Meter is ratified as a treaty by the Senate and signed by President Rutherford B. Hayes.
1890	Metric standards are received in the United States.
1893	Metric standards are declared the fundamental standards of the United States.
1954	The six primary base units are adopted: the meter, kilogram, second, ampere, Kelvin, and candela.
1960	The metric system gets its new name: *Le Systéme International d'Unités* or "S.I."
1968	Congress authorizes a study of metrication.
1975	The Metric Conversion Act of 1975 is signed by President Gerald Ford. It holds no mandatory requirements.
1988	The Omnibus Trade and Competitiveness Act amends the Metric Conversion Act. It establishes the metric system as the "preferred" system and made each federal agency responsible for implementing the metric system by the end of fiscal 1992.
1991	President George Bush issues Executive Order 12770, "Metric Usage in Federal Government Programs." It shifts the responsibility of federal metrication to the Secretary of Commerce.
1994	Fair Packaging and Labeling Act amended, requiring both customary and metric units on all consumer products.

between them? This chapter explores the history of these two systems and what is being done to add uniformity to the systems of measurement in the United States. See Table 6.1 for an overview of the major historical milestones of the metric system.

The Basics

Weights and measures are expressed in units. If I tell you, "I'm going to run a distance of five," it would have little meaning. However, when I tell you, "I'm going to run a distance of five kilometers," the statement is precise. In the latter statement, the kilometer is the *unit*. A **unit** is a precisely specified quantity of which the magnitudes or measures of other quantities of the same kind can be stated. In other words, it is a home base used for comparison. Most of us are familiar with and use many units every day: the liter, gram, yard, pound, and gallon, to name but a few. Just giving a unit a name is not enough; each of the units must be defined accurately so people in different states or even other countries have the same meaning. Standards must be established. A **standard** is any established *model* for the measurement of extent, quantity, quality, or value. The United States, for example, uses the international prototype kilogram, a cylinder made of a platinum-iridium alloy, as the standard for mass. The standard for length is the meter. It is the length of the path of a specific lightwave in a vacuum during a time interval of 1/299 792 458 of a second. It wasn't always this complicated.

Early Systems

Primitive man and ancient civilizations used crude methods to measure. Early Babylonian and Egyptian records and the Bible indicate that the width of a tribal leader's thumb (from which has come the inch) or a ruler's hand, forearm, or finger was used to mark off lengths. The weights of shells or sacred stones were used to measure weight. Then, about five or six thousand years ago, self-sufficient city-states surrounded by farms began to develop in the river valleys of the Tigris, Euphrates, Indus, and Nile rivers. As these city-states developed specialized trades, more accurate, reliable, and uniform methods of measurement were needed. A leader's hand or foot was no longer reliable. More uniformity was needed, and so, **customary** or commonly practiced systems began to develop.

In some systems the weight of kernels of grain became the standard to measure weight. For example, the unit "carat" used in measuring gems originates from the carob seed. For length or distance, a special length of wood or metal would be chosen as the standard. The standard was kept in a secure location such as a palace or temple. As trade increased and city-states grew into empires, the demand for even more accurate, precise, and uniform measurements continued to develop. The science of mathematics made it possible

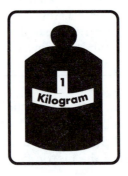

Chapter 6 / Systems of Measurement: An Historical Perspective

to create whole new systems of measurement that were suited to trade and commerce. This development occurred as empires began to navigate the seas. It was not just navigation that required this development, but all areas of science and commerce began to embark on an interdependent and symbiotic relationship that persists to this day.

The Romans

When the Roman Empire began to dominate the world, it adopted the customary system in use at the time with some divisions and modifications of its own. The Roman Empire's use of Latin contributed to some of the abbreviations and terminology in use today. The Romans divided the foot and the pound into 12 equal parts. They developed the troy pound for coins. The abbreviation for pound (lb) comes from the Latin *libra* meaning "scales." The word *mile* comes from the Latin *mille passus,* meaning "a thousand paces." This system spread through the entire Roman Empire and areas under its influence, which included most of Europe. Then, during the downfall of the Roman Empire and beyond, customary systems of measurement developed independently and along regional lines based on the old system. Western civilization would not see even so much as an attempt at such uniformity in systems of measurement until toward the end of the eighteenth century.

The French and the Metric System

The metric system derives its name from the Greek word *metron,* which means "a measure." Gabriel Mouton, vicar of St. Paul's Church in Lyon, France, is credited with being the founder and father of the metric system in 1670. (See Table 6.1.) His ideas were formed in the same period that the seeds of the French Revolution were being sown. His idea of a system of measurement had two simple principles. The first principle emphasized a decimal system. The second principle declared a single base unit of length. This base unit of length would then be used to formulate other units of measurement. For example, the base unit of volume would be calculated by making a cube from the base unit of length. The base unit for mass would be determined by filling this base unit of volume with water. For a base unit of time, a pendulum would be created that would swing the distance of the base unit of length. These ideas simmered until the French Revolution.

Our abbreviation for pound (lb) comes from the Latin *libra* meaning "scales."

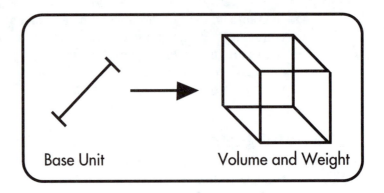

Base Unit   Volume and Weight

It was during the reign of King Louis XVI, a weak king struggling to save his country and kingdom, that Mouton's ideas began to develop into the metric system that we know today. The French Revolution was in full swing. Charles Maurice de Talleyrand-Perigord introduced a plan very similar to Mouton's to the National Assembly of France. The National Assembly was the group of revolting "common people," low-ranking clergy, and a few nobles who initiated the revolution and controlled government. Talleyrand was a French aristocrat who was bishop of Autun. He would later resign his office as bishop and become one of the foremost diplomatic figures in Europe and a famous French statesman. With changes occurring in all areas of government, it was only fitting that systems of measurement be modernized and uniform.

The English were invited to participate in the generation of this new system of measurement. However, it was not so long ago (1750s and 1760s) that the French and English had been involved in a showdown over the North American continent. The English had won the Seven Years' War, but shortly after, conceded to rebel colonists who had been funded partially by the French. Now the English were being invited by a rebel French government to work together on a scientific project. They very diplomatically declined. In April 1790, the National Assembly of France empowered the French Academy of Sciences to develop a new system of measurement.

He who has not lived during the years around 1789
cannot know what is meant by the pleasures of life.
—Charles Maurice de Talleyrand—

Committees

The French Academy of Sciences delegated the development to committees and in 1790 selected a decimal system. In 1791 the definition of a unit of length was defined as a unit equal to one ten-millionth of the distance on the surface of the Earth, from the North Pole to the equator. The new unit would be called the *metre,* which is French for the Greek *metron* meaning "a measure." It was also decided to follow Mouton's ideas for volume and mass. No decision on a measurement of time was made at this point. In 1795 France officially adopted the metric system.

Since there are irregularities to the Earth, some work was needed to make an accurate measurement for this new unit of length. Spain assisted with the actual measurement of the Earth's meridian through Barcelona, Spain, and Dunkirk, France. With this measurement and some astronomical observations, a numeration of the length of that meridian from pole to equator was established. In 1798 a standard was created. Later, in 1799, final definitions were worked out, and the construction of standards was completed. Now foreign minister, Talleyrand invited the European countries to review the work and participate in its adoption. Twelve nations attended. The United States was not invited.

Problems

There were still some problems to work out over time. Water with impurities and at differing temperatures will change its weight and volume. What about the measurement of time, temperature, and so on? These issues were still not resolved. Then in 1812, when Napoleon Bonaparte became dictator, he issued a decree allowing the use of the customary units again. This added even more difficulty for those trying to establish uniformity in measurement. Confusion reigned with measurements for 25 years.

The new system of weights and measures will be a stumbling block and the source of difficulties for several generations . . . It's just tormenting the people with trivia!!
—Napoleon I—

Acceptance

The French Assembly passed a strong act requiring the metric system to be mandatory in January 1840. The act forbid any other system to be used in France. Slowly, other nations began to accept its simple practicality. By the mid-nineteenth century, Greece, Spain, and the Netherlands had adopted the metric system. By 1880, 17 countries officially adopted it, and by the twentieth century, 35 countries had approved and were using the metric system.

The **Diplomatic Conference on the Meter** was held in Paris beginning on March 1, 1875. Twenty nations including the United States attended. The result was an agreement called the **Convention of the Meter** known as the "Treaty of the Meter." A governing body was elected. The General Conference on Weights and Measures was given authority for all actions. An International Committee of Weights and Measures was elected for administration and investigation purposes for the General Conference. The metric system was internationally accepted.

Changes

In England, the British Association for the Advancement of the Sciences (BAAS) adopted a centimeter, gram, and second (CGS) unit system to help meet the needs of science. It used the Paris meter as the standard to add centimeters, grams, and seconds as units. This system fostered the use of the unit "cc." The centimeter cubed or cubic centimeter (cc) became the measurement of volume. The BAAS made other changes that resulted in the adoption of the ampere as the base unit of quantity for electrical current.

A New Name

By 1954 six base units—meter, kilogram, second, ampere, Kelvin degree, and candela—were defined and adopted by the International Committee of Weights and Measures. These are still the primary official units today. In 1960 the entire system was named *Le Systéme International d'Unités* or the International System of Units. It is more commonly referred to by its French abbreviation "S.I." In 1971 the mole was added to the S.I. as the unit for the amount of substance. Notice that the liter is not a base unit for volume. Officially, the cubic meter is the base measure of volume for the S.I. The liter (1 cubic decimeter), although not an official S.I. unit for volume, is commonly used to measure fluid volume and is approved in the United States.

The United States and Systems of Measurement

When the metric system was being introduced in France, the United States was ratifying the Constitution. By this time, half the colonies were already 150 years old. Settlers brought their measurement practices with them from their home countries and had been using them for many years. Their measurements originated in a variety of cultures: Roman, Anglo-Saxon, Norman-French, and so on. Sweeping changes in systems of measurement would not be easy.

Before the Constitution was even ratified, Congress was already working on money. In 1786, Congress established a decimal system of coinage. There was still widespread use of the differing customary systems. Money was important even to the Founding Fathers of our government, so in 1790, President George Washington expressed a need for uniformity. Thomas Jefferson, Secretary of State, was asked to prepare a monetary plan for Congress. He presented two plans. One was based on the customary systems currently used and how to make them more uniform. The second elaborated on the decimal system of coinage that had been approved in 1786. It was basically an extension of that plan. Jefferson had played a leading role in the development of this second plan. Guess which one he supported? Of course, the second plan. He had helped develop it. Why didn't Jefferson just use the metric system?

The French metric system would not be considered for three reasons. First, the basic standard from which the tools of measurement would be

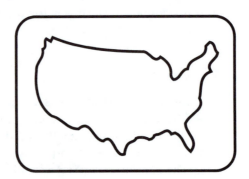

drafted was overseas in Europe. Second, the new U.S. government had not been invited to the elaborate diplomatic ceremonies surrounding the introduction of the metric system. In addition, England, to which there were still close ties, remained aloof to the idea of the metric system (most probably because of past diplomatic relations).

So, in 1792, the Mint Act was passed, which implemented the decimal system for coinage, but Congress was slow to act on a system of weights and measures. The individual states were on their own. They had to incorporate regulations into their own legal systems while they waited for a system of measurement. They had a long wait.

Metric Comes to the United States

A strange twisting of events introduced the metric system into the United States. The French had given the European delegates an iron copy of the platinum meter prototype that had been constructed for the French archives. The delegate from Switzerland, Johann George Talles, gave his copy to his friend and fellow scientist, Ferdinand Rudolf Hassler. Hassler immigrated to the United States in 1805 and brought the French standard copy with him. He was commissioned by the U.S. Coast and Geodetic Survey (the government's mapmakers) to conduct the Survey of the Coast of 1807. He used his meter as the standard. The survey was a reference for over 80 years.

Weights and measures may be ranked among the necessaries of life to every individual of human society.
—John Quincy Adams—

Why Not Metric?

With a metric standard now in the United States, why didn't the government just go ahead and start converting? In addition to most of the people using a customary method of measurement, in 1814, a bronze bar inlaid with a silver scale was brought to the United States from England. It had belonged to an instrument maker called Troughton of England. A selected part of the 82-inch bar was taken to be a 36-inch equal to the British yard, so it was used as a standard.

Then in 1817, John Quincy Adams, Secretary of State, submitted a new report to Congress. The report considered the metric system. But since Napoleon's decree a few years earlier, no one was certain what might happen to the metric system. In addition, Adams emphasized practical considerations in his report. There was already some uniformity in the states. Adams believed that this was not a time for innovation, but a time to work toward more uniformity by defining a system of measurement in terms of the British standard.

When fire broke out in the House of Parliament in Britain in 1834, its standard was lost. The United States now had no real way of knowing if the Troughton Standard was indeed accurate. When the British completed the construction of new standards in 1855, two copies of the yard and one of the avoirdupois pound were presented to the United States. The United

States had been using a troy pound as a standard for weight and opted to keep it. The new yard, however, replaced the Troughton standard. Also, a controversy surrounding custom house scales erupted, and Congress instructed the Secretary of State to supply each state with a complete set of weights and measures. Of course, the practical customary system in place was used. By the mid-nineteenth century, the United States was already committed to an obsolete standard and system.

The Conversion Begins

Congress established the National Academy of Sciences in 1863, and scientists were involved with weights and measures right away. Scientists pushed to legalize the metric system so they could work in harmony with other scientists around the world. In just three years, the president signed a bill legalizing the use of the metric system in the United States for any purpose. The bill didn't have much punch, but like most of their associates in other countries, scientists could now legally use the metric system.

> By adopting the metric system, which is the international standard of measurement, we can improve our competitiveness and our ability to sell our products in world markets.
> **—Gary P. Carver—**

After the United States participated in the Diplomatic Conference on the Meter in 1875, U.S. scientists became intimately involved with the supervision of the construction of the new metric system standards in France. By 1893 the new metric standards were declared fundamental standards of measurement for the United States. The use of new standards didn't change measurements in everyday life because the metric system wasn't required; the meter was just being used as the standard to define everything else. By 1878, the Convention of the Meter was ratified by the Senate as a treaty and signed by President Rutheford B. Hayes. By the end of the nineteenth century, the United States had adopted the metric system as legal and science was widely using it. There was, however, still discrepancy as far as business and commerce were concerned.

It wasn't until the mid-twentieth century that more definite efforts at uniformity and conversion were made. In 1959, representatives from different countries, including the United States, refined conversions between systems, and then in 1960 the metric system was renamed *Le Systéme International d'Unités* or "S.I." As debates both for and against conversion continued, Congress ordered a study in 1968 that ended in 1971. The National Bureau of Standards (now the National Institute of Standards and Technology) report was titled "A Metric America: A Decision Whose Time Has Come." The study cited that the United States was already metric in some respects and was becoming more so. It recommended that Congress pass legislation that would provide for this process to go forward over a 10-year period. The report contributed to the passage of the **Metric Conversion Act of 1975.** It was signed into law by President Gerald Ford. The act stated, "the policy of the United States shall be to coordinate and plan the increasing use of the

Metric System in the United States and to establish a U.S. Metric Board to coordinate the voluntary conversion to the metric system." President Jimmy Carter appointed the 17-member board. The Metric Conversion Act raised the expectation of a 10-year voluntary transition to the metric system. However, no mandatory time requirements were enacted, and it lacked a clear objective. Much of the American public ignored the efforts of the Metric Board. The Board reported to Congress that it did not possess the necessary mandates to bring about conversion. President Ronald Reagan dissolved it in 1982 when efforts to reduce federal spending became a central public issue.

World Trade

Conversion slowed over the next few years and Congress recognized that world trade could be hampered if American commerce did not conform to world standards. **Metrication,** converting to the metric system, of America was becoming imperative to world economic survival. The United States was the only industrialized nation not metricized. Market preferences in the European Common Market and the expanding Pacific Rim are metric. "Worldclass" products would need to be produced in order to remain competitive in the international marketplace. Congress responded by passing the **Omnibus Trade and Competitiveness Act of 1988.** It was an amendment to the Metric Conversion Act. It designated the metric system as the "preferred system of weights and measures for United States trade and commerce." The legislation also made each federal agency responsible for implementing metric usage in grants, contracts, and other business-related activities. The goal was to have the federal government metricized by the end of fiscal year 1992. Unfortunately, there was no statutory provisions made for leadership or coordination.

On July 25, 1991, President George Bush issued Executive Order 12770, "Metric Usage in Federal Government Programs." The order gave the Secretary of Commerce the authority to lead and coordinate the implementation of the metric conversions required by the Omnibus Trade Act. The responsibility was delegated to the Under Secretary for Technology, with staff support from the Office of Metric Programs and the National Institute of Standards and Technology (NIST). An annual report from the Secretary of Commerce to the president must include an assessment of progress toward the goal of metrication.

The Metric Conversion Act, its amendments, and the executive order apply directly only to the federal government. Business and commerce are indirectly affected. The law does not require that business convert to the metric system. Foreign competition might even prefer that American companies not convert. However, to remain a major world force in a global economy, businesses immediately began converting. Most science and medicine-related industries converted a long time ago. Those businesses that operate through federal contracts, loans, and grants will have to begin making the conversion to the metric system to serve a government almost completely metric.

In 1994, the Fair Packaging and Labeling Act was amended by the Food and Drug Administration (FDA) to require the use of both customary and metric units on all consumer products.

As metrication continues, understanding the old U.S. Customary Weights and Measures System and learning the metric system may still be necessary. Some industries and the general population may still be using all or parts of the old customary system, so conversions between the two systems may still be required.

EXERCISE 6.1 SYSTEMS OF MEASUREMENT

(Answers may be found in Appendix C.)

1. The U.S. Constitution gives _____ the power to set the standard for weights and measures in the United States.

    a. president
    b. Congress
    c. Omnibus Trade Act
    d. General Conference on Weights and Measures

2. A precisely specified quantity of which the magnitudes or measures of other quantities of the same kind can be stated; a home base used for comparison is a:

    a. unit
    b. standard
    c. weight
    d. none of the above

3. Any established model for the measurement of extent, quantity, quality, or value is a:

    a. unit
    b. standard
    c. weight
    d. none of the above

4. Commonly practiced systems of measurement are also known as:

    a. Babylonian systems
    b. metric systems
    c. Roman systems
    d. customary systems

5. The founder and father of the metric system is:

    a. Charles Maurice de Talleyrand-Perigord
    b. Gabriel Mouton
    c. Napoleon I
    d. none of the above

6. The metric system originated in

    a. the United States
    b. England
    c. France
    d. Spain

7. The word *meter* is derived from the Greek *metron* meaning:

    a. a distance
    b. a measure
    c. a weight
    d. a system

8. The Diplomatic Conference on the Meter held in 1875 resulted in an agreement known as the:

    a. Convention of the Meter or the "Treaty of the Meter"
    b. Paris Convention of Weights and Measures
    c. Treaty of Weights and Measures
    d. Treaty of the Metric System

9. The United States did not attend the Diplomatic Conference on the Meter.

    a. True
    b. False

10. *Le Systéme International d'Unités,* the International System of Units, is commonly referred to as:

    a. "I.S.U."
    b. "S.I."
    c. "The System"
    d. none of the above

11. The United States did not convert to the metric system in the late 1700s and early 1800s because of close ties to England and:

    a. scientists were opposed to the idea
    b. the National Assembly of Sciences opposed the idea
    c. most people used a customary system of measurement
    d. the president had signed a law banning the metric system

12. The legislation that was passed in the late 1980s and began true conversion to the metric system in the United States is the:

    a. Metric Conversion Act
    b. Omnibus Trade and Competitiveness Act
    c. World Trade Act
    d. Metric America Act

13. When President George Bush issued Executive Order 12770 in 1991, it ultimately gave _____ the responsibility to coordinate metrication.

    a. Congress
    b. General Conference on Weights and Measures
    c. French Assembly
    d. Secretary of Commerce

14. Practical staff support for metrication comes from:

    a. Congress
    b. Office of Metric Programs
    c. National Institute of Standards and Technology (NIST)
    d. Both b and c

15. This legislation required the use of both customary and metric units on all consumer products:

    a. Metric Conversion Act
    b. Fair Packaging and Labeling Act
    c. Omnibus Trade and Competitiveness Act
    d. World Trade Act

The U.S. Customary Weights and Measures System

OBJECTIVES

In order to work dosage calculation problems as an emergency health care provider, you should be able to:

1. Identify a definition of the U.S. customary weights and measures system.

2. Identify a definition of the apothecary system.

3. Recognize and utilize selected units of the apothecary system.

4. Recognize and utilize Roman numerals.

5. Recognize and utilize Arabic numerals.

6. Identify a definition of the avoirdupois system.

7. Recognize and utilize selected units of the avoirdupois system.

8. Identify a definition of the household system.

9. Recognize and utilize selected units of the household system.

10. Utilize the factor method for conversions.

11. Convert between the apothecary, the avoirdupois, and the household systems of measurement.

INTRODUCTION

- *What is the difference between Roman numerals and Arabic numerals?*
- *How many systems make up the U.S. system?*
- *What's the difference between an apothecary and an avoirdupois pound?*

Because of the wonderful diversity of cultures here, the United States has been referred to both as a melting pot and a tossed salad. Those two analogies also apply to the old system of measurement: the U.S. Customary Weights and Measures System. Many different people from many lands brought not only their cultures and languages, but their systems of measurement as well. Since there is a significant number of laypeople still using this system, a brief review and some practice is in order.

> *I have often admired the mystical ways of Pythagoras,*
> *and the secret magic of numbers.*
> **—Sir Thomas Brown—**

7.1 THE U.S. CUSTOMARY WEIGHTS AND MEASURES SYSTEM

The old U.S. Customary Weights and Measures System, or the customary system, is an outdated system of measurement with irregularities between units. Look at the relationship between the units of distance: 12 inches equals 1 foot, 3 feet equals 1 yard, 1760 yards equals 1 mile, and so on. The relationships are based on tradition, not on a logical system. Health care professionals should not be using it. However, parts of the system are still in use by the general public. For example, when someone asks you, "How much do you weigh?" inevitably the units in the answer will be pounds, not kilograms. The apothecaries' system, the avoirdupois system, the troy system of weight, and the household system are all components of the old U.S. customary system.

The Apothecary System

The word "apothecary" originates from the Greek word *apotheke* which means a storing place. In England and Ireland it refers to a physician and dispenser of drugs who is licensed by the Society of Apothecaries' of London or the Apothecaries' Hall of Ireland. In the United States, the term apothecary is declining in use. It refers to a pharmacist or a pharmacy. The apothecaries' weights and measures system is one of the oldest of the drug measurement systems that was used by physicians and pharmacists. It is commonly referred to as the apothecaries' system.

TABLE 7.1 Apothecaries' Measure

FLUID MEASURE

60 minims (Mx or ♏)	= 1 fluid dram
8 fluid drams (fl dr or ʒ)	= 1 fluid ounce
16 fluid ounces (fl oz or ℥)	= 1 pint
2 pints (fl pt)	= 1 quart
4 quarts (qt)	= 1 gallon

WEIGHT

20 grains (gr)	= 1 scruple
60 grains	= 1 dram
480 grains	= 1 ounce
5760 grains	= 1 lb ap
3 scruples (s or Э)	= 1 dram
24 scruples	= 1 oz
288 scruples	= 1 pound (lb ap)
8 drams	= 1 ounce or 480 grains
96 drams	= 1 lb ap
12 ounces	= 1 pound (lb ap)

Units

The units of the apothecaries' system are no longer recommended for use by medical professionals. Some instructors and institutions may still require the student to be familiar with some of the units of this system. See Table 7.1 for a table of the units of fluid and weight measurement. A more complete table of the U.S. customary system (Table 7.4) is provided at the end of this chapter. Later, in Chapter 9, conversions between selected apothecary units and metric units will be discussed.

Roman Numerals

Since the apothecaries' system arose out of the Greco-Roman tradition, it uses Roman numerals and places. Most emergency care providers are more familiar with Arabic numbers. Even though these units are obsolete, Roman numerals are sometimes used in medical documentation. Being familiar with some simplified rules will help.

The symbol for one (i) and five (v) are often written in lowercase with a line and a dot over the symbol for one. They can also be written in capitals. There is good reason to use lowercase. This practice originated because ink on parchment used at the time would "bleed," causing some confusion. Nowadays, just sloppy penmanship and small blanks on forms can cause problems. A one used as a capital (I) can run together or be easily confused with other symbols. The dot helps keep the one(s) (i̇) distinct from other numbers. The number IV could easily be mistaken for III when handwritten. Using lowercase (i̇v̄) helps to avoid misperceptions and errors.

When using apothecaries' abbreviations and Roman numerals, the abbreviation of a symbol is written *before* the quantity. For example, "gr. v" is 5 grains, "♏ LX" is 60 minims. When abbreviations are not used, Arabic numbers are used before the apothecary unit. For example: 5 grains, 2 drams, and so on. Quantities of less than one are expressed as common fractions. The symbol gr $\frac{1}{4}$ means one-quarter grain. The fraction $\frac{1}{2}$ is not written as a fraction, however. It is written as "$\overline{ss}$," for example; "gr $\overline{ss}$" is $\frac{1}{2}$ of a grain.

The Roman numerals and their values are:

i or (î) or I = 1	C = 100
v or V = 5	D = 500
x or X = 10	M = 1000
L = 50	$\overline{ss} = \frac{1}{2}$

When a letter/symbol of smaller value is placed first, the value is subtracted (îv or IV = 5 − 1 = 4). When a letter of larger value is placed first, the value is added (vi or VI = 5 + 1 = 6). Repeating a letter repeats its value (XX = 20).

Avoirdupois System of Measure

The avoirdupois system of measure originates from the French *avoir de pois,* which, translated very loosely, means "goods (sold by) of weight."(See Table 7.2.) This system was designed to measure coarse and heavy articles. All measures of capacity are cubic measures. When the apothecaries' and avoirdupois systems are compared (See Table 7.4), we find still another reason that the customary system is just difficult and illogical. Look at the number of ounces in an avoirdupois pound (16 oz = 1 lb avdp). Now look at the number of ounces in the apothecary system (12 oz = 1 lb ap). Same system, different values. Very confusing.

NOTE: The avoirdupois pound (16 oz = 1 lb avdp) is the fundamental unit of weight in the customary system.

Troy Weight

The troy weight system measures precious metals and gems such as gold and silver. It is not used in emergency settings.

The Household System

Many of the liquid measurements of the household system are identical to those of the apothecaries' system. (See Table 7.3.) However, not all house-

TABLE 7.2 Avoirdupois Measure

WEIGHT

16 drams	= 1 ounce
1 ounce	= 437.5 grains
16 ounces	= 1 pound (avdp)
1 pound	= 7000 grains

TABLE 7.3 General or Household Measure*

FLUID MEASURE

60 drops	= 1 teaspoon (tsp)
3 teaspoons	= 1 tablespoon (tbsp)
2 tablespoons	= 1 ounce
8 ounces	= 1 cup
2 cups (16 ounces)	= 1 pint

*Household measures are not precise. Do not substitute household equivalents for medication prescribed by a physician.

hold droppers and teaspoons are alike. Therefore, this system cannot be relied upon by health care professionals. However, some patients and families, especially elderly patients, use this system to measure liquid medications since they most likely grew up with it. Being familiar with this system may help you when you encounter patients using it.

Conversion Factors

Each of the systems of measurement is divided into units of length, area, volume, weight, liquid capacity, and so on. Emergency care providers will be primarily concerned with liquid capacity, weight, and to a lesser degree, length. Each of these measures in each system will have a fundamental unit. It may become necessary to convert from one measured quantity to another within a system or to convert between systems (conversions between the customary system and the metric system will be discussed in Chapter 9, Conversions Between Systems).

Conversions can be performed using a **conversion factor.** A conversion factor is a multiplier consisting of two or more units used to convert one quantity into a second quantity having different units. The use of conversion factors is called the **factor unit method** because the factor is numerically equivalent to one. A step-by-step method used to convert either within or between systems is utilized in the pages ahead.

Factor Unit Method

Example: A football field is 100 yards long. How many feet are in that field?

1. Examine the information. Determine what unit (system) is given and what unit (system) is being sought:

    yards (customary) → feet (customary)

2. Write down the information with the given information to the left of an equal sign (that will be multiplied by a conversion factor) and the desired unknown units to the right of the equal sign:

    100 yards × factor = ? feet

3. Choose the conversion factor that eliminates the given unit (system) and results in the unit (system) being sought. Tables are provided in various chapters and Appendix F. A table states that 1 yard is equal to 3 feet. A conversion factor can be written in one of two ways based on this fact. The first conversion factor, F_1, can express 1 yard equals 3 feet:

$$F_1 = \frac{1 \text{ yd}}{3 \text{ ft}}$$

Expressing 3 feet equals 1 yard can be expressed as F_2:

$$F_2 = \frac{3 \text{ ft}}{1 \text{ yd}}$$

F_2 will eliminate the yards and result in feet.

4. Work the arithmetic:

$$100 \text{ yards} \times \text{factor} = ? \text{ feet}$$

becomes

$$100 \text{ yd} \times \frac{3 \text{ ft}}{1 \text{ yd}} = ? \text{ feet}$$

The unit *yards* cancel out.

$$100 \times \frac{3 \text{ ft}}{1} = ? \text{ ft}$$
$$300 \text{ ft} = ? \text{ ft}$$

Conversion factors are expressed in tables/charts or as fractions as above. When Chapter 9, Conversions Between Systems, is discussed, you may want to return to this discussion to help with the conversions.

In the following tables, the fundamental unit is defined and relative values provided. Conversion charts are provided in Chapter 9.

The U. S. Customary System

TABLE 7.4 Tables of Weights and Measures

Adapted from the New Standard Encyclopedias

LENGTH	LIQUID CAPACITY
The fundamental unit of length is the yard. It is defined as 0.9144 of the length of the "S.I." meter	The fundamental unit is the gallon. It is defined as the volume of 231 cubic inches.

GENERAL UNITS		APOTHECARIES' FLUID MEASURE	
12 inches (in., or ″)	= 1 foot	60 minims (min)	= 1 fluid dram
3 feet (ft, or ′)	= 1 yard	8 fluid drams (fl dr)	= 1 fluid ounce
1 yard (yd)	= 36 in	16 fluid ounces (fl oz)	= 1 fluid pint
1760 yd/5280 ft	= 1 mile (mi)	2 fluid pints (fl pt)	= 1 fluid quart (32 fl oz)
		4 liquid quarts (liq qt)	= 1 gallon (8 pt, 128 fl oz)

HOUSEHOLD UNITS	
60 drops (gtt)	= 1 teaspoon (t)
3 teaspoons (t)	= 1 tablespoon
2 tablespoons (T)	= 1 oz
8 oz	= 1 cup
2 cups/16 oz	= 1 liquid pint
2 pints	= 1 quart (qt)

WEIGHT

The fundamental unit of weight is the avoirdupois pound. It is defined as 0.453 592 37 of the weight of the international prototype kilogram.

AVOIRDUPOIS	
16 drams (dr avdp)	= 1 ounce (oz)
16 ounces (oz avdp)	= 1 pound (lb avdp)
2000 pounds (lb avdp)	= 1 ton

APOTHECARIES'	
20 grains (gr ap)	= 1 scruple
3 scruples (s ap)	= 1 dram
8 drams (dr ap)	= 1 ounce
12 ounces (oz ap)	= 1 pound (lb ap)
1 pound (lb ap)	= $\frac{144}{175}$ lb avdp
60 grains	= 1 dram
480 grains	= 1 ounce
5760 grains	= 1 pound (lb ap)
288 scruples	= 1 pound (lb ap)
96 drams	= 1 pound (lb ap)

(Answers may be found in Appendix C.)

Express the following in Roman numerals:

1. 4 = _____

2. 6 = _____

3. 9 = _____

4. 7 = _____

5. 30 = _____

Express the following in Arabic numbers:

6. ii = _____

7. iv = _____

8. ix = _____

9. xix = _____

10. xxiv = _____

Convert between the following customary units:

11. fl pt i̅ = ℥ _____ = ʒ _____

12. fl ʒ LXi̅v̅ (64) = ℥ _____ = fl pt _____

13. gr LX (60) = Э _____ = ʒ _____

14. ℔ 240 = Э _____ = fl oz ap _____

15. ʒ XCv̅i̅ (96) = ℥ _____ = lb ap _____

16. 1 lb ap = gr ap _____

17. 1 lb avdp = gr avpd _____

18. 1 lb ap = oz ap _____

19. 1 lb avpd = oz avpd _____

20. 1 tbsp = _____ tsp

The Metric System

OBJECTIVES

In order to work dosage calculation problems as an emergency health care provider, you should be able to:

1. Identify a definition of the metric system.

2. Identify the seven base units of the metric system.

3. Recognize and utilize the common multiples, submultiples, and prefixes of the metric system.

4. Utilize the metric system under the rules of the U.S. government's National Institute of Standards and Technology.

5. Convert between the units of the metric system.

INTRODUCTION

- *Is the liter a unit of the metric system?*
- *What does the prefix "kilo" mean?*
- *Are commas really not used anymore?*

Many people have expressed anxiety about learning or relearning a new system of measurement. It is reassuring to know that the metric system is very logical and practical—just like most emergency care providers! That's probably why most emergency care providers have little trouble understanding it. If you need a review, or if it's totally unfamiliar to you, this chapter will get you on track. There are plenty of problems for you to practice.

> *Most people would die sooner than think;*
> *in fact, they do so.*
> **—Bertrand Russell—**

8.1 THE METRIC SYSTEM

The International System of Units, or more commonly, the metric system, is abbreviated SI (from the French *Le Systéme International d'Unités*). It is an international system of measurement governed by the General Conference on Weights and Measures and is administered by the International Committee of Weights and Measures. It provides a logical and international system of measurement for science, industry, and commerce. It is regulated in the United States through the Secretary of Commerce and may be modified and defined by the National Institute of Standards and Technology.

Prefixes

The metric system is a decimal system that is based on multiples of 10. Multiples larger than the base unit are expressed in multiples of 10, and those smaller than the base units are expressed in decimal fractions that are submultiples of 10. Greek prefixes are used to express these multiples and submultiples. Prefixes produce units that are of an appropriate size for the application needed. For example, the centimeter could be used to measure body dimensions, the meter for measuring short distances, and the kilometer for measuring long distances. Adding the prefix kilo, which means a thousand, to the unit gram can be used to denote 1000 grams. Thus, 1000 grams becomes 1 kilogram. Unlike the U.S. customary system, it does not require complicated conversions from unit to unit. Simply moving the decimal point is all that is needed. Some prefixes are used more frequently than others, and some are very rarely used. When using prefixes, only one should be used at a time. Prefix symbols for values over a million or greater are capitalized, and those symbols for values below a million are written in lowercase. See Table 8.1 for the most common multiples, submultiples, and prefixes.

Units of the Metric System

The metric system has seven base units: the meter for length, the second for time, the ampere for electric current, the candela for luminous intensity, the Kelvin for temperature, the kilogram for mass, and the mole for amount of substance. There are two supplementary units: the radian and steradian used to measure angles. All other SI units, such as the hertz, degree Celsius, or the newton, are derived from these base units. Noticeably lacking is the liter. The SI unit for volume is the cubic meter. The liter, although not an SI unit, is an approved and preferred unit of volume because of its practical importance in

TABLE 8.1 Common Multiples, Submultiples, and Prefixes

MULTIPLES AND SUBMULTIPLES	PREFIX NAME	PREFIX SYMBOL
$1\,000\,000\,000\,000 = 10^{12}$	tera	T
$1\,000\,000\,000 = 10^{9}$	giga	G
$1\,000\,000 = 10^{6}$	mega	M
$1\,000 = 10^{3}$	kilo	k
$100 = 10^{2}$	hecto	h
$10 = 10^{1}$	deka	da
$1 = 10^{0}$	**Base Unit**	
$0.1 = 10^{-1}$	deci	d
$0.01 = 10^{-2}$	centi	c
$0.001 = 10^{-3}$	milli	m
$0.000\,001 = 10^{-6}$	micro	μ
$0.000\,000\,001 = 10^{-9}$	nano	n
$0.000\,000\,000\,001 = 10^{-12}$	pico	p

Europe and the United States. There are other nonmetric units that are acceptable to use in the United States such as the minute, the hour, and the nautical mile. In addition to the rules regarding prefixes and units, there are other important rules that are sometimes not explained in typical high school or college math courses. To have excellent documentation, you will want to be familiar with and use the rules set forth by the federal government.

8.2 RULES TO THE METRIC SYSTEM

Capitals

Units. Unless beginning a sentence, the names of all units start with lowercase letters. The units meter, gram, liter, and so on begin with lowercase letters. There is one exception, however. When using "degree Celsius," the unit "degree" is lowercase, but the word "Celsius" is capitalized. Written normal body temperature would, for example, appear as:

37 degrees Celsius

Table 8.2 lists the most common metric units and symbols. It also demonstrates the use of some common multiples and submultiples and their symbols.

Symbols. Generally, the metric unit symbols are written in lowercase letters, for example, "km" for kilometer or "mg" for milligram. Since the liter is not an SI unit, it is set apart. The symbol for liter is capitalized. If a unit name is derived from a person's name, it is also capitalized. For example,

L for liter

Pa for Pascal

mL for milliliter

Plurals

Units. The names of units (meter, gram, etc.) are only made plural when the numerical value that precedes them is more than one. The

TABLE 8.2 Common Metric Unit Names/Symbols

BASE UNIT	NAME	SYMBOL
length	kilometer	km
	meter	m
	centimeter	cm
	millimeter	mm
weight	kilogram	kg
	gram	g
	milligram	mg
volume	liter	L
	milliliter	mL
pressure	kilopascal	kPa
	pascal	Pa

only exception to this rule is when zero degrees Celsius is used. For example,

3 liters or 0.5 liter *not* 0.5 liters

$\frac{1}{2}$ liter *not* $\frac{1}{2}$ liters

NOTE: Since the metric system is a decimal system, decimal fractions are preferred over common fractions.

Symbols. Symbols for units are not pluralized. For example,

50 mL = 50 milliliters

50 mL *not* 50 mL's

Spacing

Spaces. A space is used in between the number and the symbol for which it refers. For example,

10 k, 120 kg, 37° C

Hyphens. Hyphens do not need to be used between a number and a metric unit when used as a one-thought modifier. However, if a hyphen *is* used, the name of the metric value should be written out. For example,

a 1-liter bag *not* a 1-L bag

a 10-kilometer run *not* a 10-k run or a 10-km run

Commas. Some countries use commas where we use periods. Therefore, spaces, not commas, are used when writing metric values containing *five* or more digits. For values with *four* digits, either a space or no space is acceptable. The spaces are added either side of the decimal point. For example,

1 234 567 km *not* 1,234,567 km

1000 km or 1 000 km

0.123 456 mm

Period

Do not use a period with metric unit names and symbols except at the end of a sentence. For example,

10 cm *not* 10 cm.

Decimal Point

The dot or period is used as the decimal point within numbers. In numbers less than one, a zero is written before the decimal point. This is especially important for health care professionals. This "leading" zero draws attention to the decimal point and helps prevent mistakes in dosage calculations. For example,

0.5 mL *not* .5 mL

Never follow a whole number with a decimal point and zero. The decimal point may not be seen, causing a potential tenfold overdose.

1 mg *not* 1.0 mg

Conversions Between Multiples. The most common multiples/prefixes used are the *kilo,* the *milli,* and the *micro.* The multiple between each unit in the metric system is 10. That is the basis of the decimal system. Between the most common multiples and prefixes, the multiple is 1000. The accompanying chart may be used to help you remember the relationship between the most common multiples or prefixes. To convert from kilograms to grams, either multiply by 1000 or move the decimal three places to the right. To convert from grams to kilograms, either divide by 1000 or move the decimal places to the left. The same principle applies between grams and milligrams and between milligrams and micrograms. The multiple between kilograms and milligrams is 1 000 000. Table 8.3 demonstrates this same principle from a different perspective.

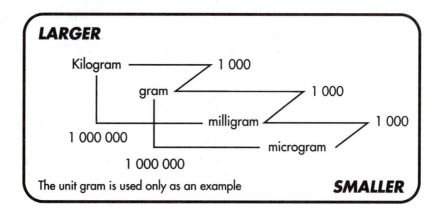

TABLE 8.3 Conversions Between Multiples

FROM:	TO:	TO CONVERT:
kilograms	grams	Multiply by 1000 or move decimal three places to the right.
grams	milligrams	Multiply by 1000 or move decimal three places to the right.
milligrams	micrograms	Multiply by 1000 or move decimal three places to the right.
kilograms	milligrams	Multiply by 1 000 000 or move decimal six places to right.
grams	micrograms	Multiply by 1 000 000 or move decimal six places to right.
micrograms	milligrams	Divide by 1000 or move decimal three places to the left.
milligrams	grams	Divide by 1000 or move decimal three places to the left.
grams	kilograms	Divide by 1000 or move decimal three places to the left.
micrograms	grams	Divide by 1 000 000 or move decimal six places to the left.
milligrams	kilograms	Divide by 1 000 000 or move decimal six places to the left.

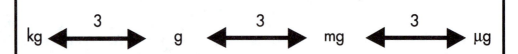

kg ←─ 3 ─→ g ←─ 3 ─→ mg ←─ 3 ─→ μg

To convert from one multiple to the other, move the decimal point three places in the direction indicated. For example, if you are converting grams to milligrams, move the decimal three places to the right. Grams are used here only as an example.

To convert from one decimal to the other, move the decimal point three places in the direction indicated. For example, if you are converting grams to milligrams, move the decimal three places to the right. Grams are used here only as an example.

There is another way to look at these relationships. Pay special attention to the relationship of milliliters, cubic centimeters, and centimeter cubed. Table 8.4 provides common conversion factors for the health care professional:

TABLE 8.4 Metric System

1000 μg = 1 mg	1000 mL = 1 L
1000 mg = 1 g	1000 L = 1 kL
1000 g = 1 kg	**1 mL = 1 cc = 1 cm³**
	1000 mm = 1 m
	100 cm = 1 m
	1000 m = 1 km

(Answers may be found in Appendix C.)

1. 1 g   = _____ mg   21. 0.8 mg   = _____ μg

2. 1 mg   = _____ μg   22. 250 mL   = _____ L

3. 7500 mg   = _____ g   23. 75 000 g   = _____ kg

4. 1600 μg   = _____ mg   24. 400 μg   = _____ mg

5. 1000 mg   = _____ g   25. 200 mg   = _____ μg

6. 0.75 g   = _____ mg   26. 1000 mg   = _____ μg

7. 500 mL   = _____ L   27. 0.000 5 g   = _____ mg

8. 0.25 L   = _____ mL   28. 10 kg   = _____ mg

9. 1.6 mg   = _____ μg   29. 0.0016 kg   = _____ mg

10. 2500 g   = _____ kg   30. 0.03 L   = _____ mL

11. 0.715 g   = _____ mg   31. 200 000 μg   = _____ mg

12. 400 000 μg   = _____ mg   32. 1000 g   = _____ kg

13. 125 mg   = _____ g   33. 600 μg   = _____ mg

14. 0.1 g   = _____ mg   34. 10 000 mg   = _____ g

15. 0.45 L   = _____ mL   35. 4 mg   = _____ g

16. 1.5 L   = _____ mL   36. 6.8 kg   = _____ g

17. 80 000 g   = _____ kg   37. 1600 μg   = _____ mg

18. 4000 mg   = _____ g   38. 0.0016 g   = _____ μg

19. 800 μg   = _____ mg   39. 1500 mL   = _____ L

20. 1000 mL   = _____ L   40. 1 μg   = _____ mg

chapter 9

Conversions Between Systems

OBJECTIVES

In order to work dosage calculation problems as an emergency health care provider, you should be able to:

1. Prepare a value with a combination of units for conversion.

2. Locate the proper conversion factor in charts or tables.

3. Convert values from differing systems of measurement.

4. Utilize the metric system rounding rules of the U.S. Government's National Institute of Standards and Technology.

5. Approximate values in an emergency using the "2 a.m. rule."

INTRODUCTION

- *How complicated are the rules of conversion?*
- *How do the government's rules of rounding differ from what I'm used to?*
- *What is the 2 a.m. rule?*

Since a lot of people are still using outdated systems of measurement, we must be prepared to convert between the "old" U.S. Customary Weights and Measures System and the metric system. After a little practice, it becomes quite easy.

Angling may be said to be so like the mathematics,
that it can never be fully learnt.
—Izaak Walton—

9.1 CONVERSIONS BETWEEN SYSTEMS

Most people are still using the customary system of weights and measures at home. Contrast this against the fact that the U.S. government, medicine, and the sciences and more and more segments of industry are using the metric system. The importance of knowing the relationships between systems cannot be overemphasized. In working problems of all types connected with drugs and solutions, it will be more practical and easier to work with quantities in the metric system. This unit provides the rules for conversion and rounding and both approximate and exact conversion factors supplied and approved by the U. S. Department of Commerce, National Institute of Standards and Technology.

Conversion

The following simplified federal standards should be used when converting and rounding metric values obtained from customary system conversions:

1. **Preparing to Convert.** If the customary value is expressed by a combination of units, such as pounds and ounces, it should first be converted to the smaller unit. For example,

$$30 \text{ lb } 2\frac{1}{2} \text{ oz} = 482.5 \text{ oz}$$

2. **Factor Conversion.** Make the calculation to convert to the metric system. Conversion factors are provided in the tables following these rules. The factor unit method is explained on pages 67–68 of Chapter 7.

NOTE: Remember that metric values are not expressed using common fractions. Metric values are expressed in decimal fractions only.

3. **Rounding the Metric Value.** Compare the metric value to the customary value. If the first significant digit of the metric value, usually a whole number, is equal to or greater than the first significant digit of the customary value, round the metric value to the same number of places or digits as there are in the customary value. For example,

4 gal $\times$ 3.785 = 15.14 L, which rounds to 15 L

The "15" in 15.14 liters is equal to or greater than the "4" in 4 gallons so the decimals are dropped in the metric conversion. If, however, the first significant digit of the metric value is smaller than the first significant digit of the customary value, round to one more significant digit. For example,

163 lb $\times$ 0.45 = 73.35 kg, which rounds to 73.4 kg

The "73" in 73.35 kilograms is smaller than the "163" in 163 pounds so the metric value is rounded to one more place than the customary value. In this case the metric value is rounded to the tenth decimal place. Standard rules of rounding are then utilized (see Section 2.1, Decimal Fraction Fundamentals, page 24).

The 2 a.m. Rule

Federal standards provide accurate conversions when precise measurements are required and time permits. Sometimes, in emergency situations, rounding is replaced with approximations in the interest of time. These approximations of the standards are referred to in street jargon as the "2 a.m. rules." When considering the use of the 2 a.m. rule, it is critical to consider the clinical or therapeutic ramifications of that decision. Most of the time those approximations may not make any difference at all. But, when considering pediatrics, geriatrics, or other special situations, approximations could affect the therapeutic ranges of the medication that is being given. So, consult your protocols, standing orders, or medical director for guidance.

Approximating

Some conversions are approximated to the nearest practical and reasonable number. Approximating is what most of us have called "rounding" in the past, but it does not necessarily follow the National Institute of Standards and Technology's rules on rounding conversions. When approximating, the number is usually, but not always, going to be a whole number. For example,

$$1.3 \text{ mL} \approx 1 \text{ mL}$$

$$3.7 \text{ mL} \approx 4 \text{ mL}$$

$$0.35 \text{ mL} \approx 0.4 \text{ ml}$$

$$67.5 \text{ kg} \approx 68 \text{ kg}$$

Weight

One of these simplifications involves the conversion of pounds to kilograms. Rather than using a federal conversion factor, the following method is used by a lot of paramedics. At first glance it might look more difficult than it actually is. It can be easily calculated in your head.

1. *Divide* the weight in pounds by 2 (remember to approximate):

$$200 \text{ lb} \div 2 \approx 100$$

2. *Multiply* by 10%:

$$100 \times 10\% \approx 10$$

3. *Subtract* the percent from the quotient and place the metric value:

$$100 - 10 = 90 \text{ kg}$$

It is important to emphasize that the 2 a.m. rule and approximating should be used only in the event of an emergency. It clearly should not replace orders, drug cards, or accurate drug dosage calculations. Conversions should always follow a rule of reason.

Conversion Factors

Conversion factors for the metric system are listed in Tables 9.1 and 9.2. The first is the format in use by the federal government. The second table may be more familiar to those who use the factor unit method. Either may be used. Choose whichever is more familiar or easy for you.

TABLE 9.1 Federal Government Format (Adapted from Federal Standard 376B, U.S. Department of Commerce)

The quantities and common medical quantities shown are grouped according to length, volume, weight (mass), pressure, and temperature. The first column is labeled **FROM.** This column lists the customary units that are used to express the quantities for that subsection. The second column, labeled **TO,** gives either the S.I. unit or other preferred units approved by the federal government. The third column, labeled **MULTIPLY BY,** gives the conversion factor (generally to seven significant digits). Multiply the number in the **FROM** column by the number in the **MULTIPLY BY** column in order to get the number in the **TO** column.

Conversion factors that are exact in the **MULTIPLY BY** column are in bold type. Accepted approximate conversion factors are in plain type in parentheses below the more exact factor.

Common Medical Quantities		
FROM CUSTOMARY LENGTH	**TO METRIC LENGTH**	**MULTIPLY BY**
inch	**centimeter (cm)**	**2.54**
	millimeter (mm)	**25.4**
foot	**meter (m)**	0.304 800 6
		(0.3)
foot	**centimeter (cm)**	30.480 06
		(30)
yard	**meter**	**0.914 4**
		(0.9)
mile	**kilometer (km)**	**1.609 344**
FROM CUSTOMARY VOLUME	**TO METRIC VOLUME**	**MULTIPLY BY**
teaspoon	**milliliter (mL)**	5
tablespoon	**milliliter (mL)**	15
fluid ounce	**milliliter (mL)**	29.573 53
		(30)
cup	**liter (L)**	0.24
pint	**liter (L)**	0.473 176 5
		(0.47)
quart	**liter (L)**	0.946 352 9
		(0.95)
gallon	**liter (L)**	3.785 412
		(3.8)

FROM CUSTOMARY WEIGHT (mass)	TO METRIC WEIGHT (mass)	MULTIPLY BY
grain	**milligram (mg)**	64.798 91 (65)
ounce, avoirdupois	**gram (g)**	28.349 52 (28)
pound	**kilogram (kg)**	**0.453 592 37** (0.45)

FROM CUSTOMARY PRESSURE	TO METRIC PRESSURE	MULTIPLY BY
millimeter of mercury	**kilopascal (kPa)**	0.133 322 4 (0.13)
torr	**pascal (Pa)**	133.322 4 (133)
pounds per square inch	**kilopascal (kPa)**	6.894 757 (6.9)

FROM CUSTOMARY TEMPERATURE	TO METRIC TEMPERATURE (exact)	MULTIPLY BY
degree Fahrenheit (°F)	**degree Celsius (°C)**	$\frac{5}{9}$ (after subtracting 32)

Note: Some older sources have two conversion factors for grains to milligrams. You may also see or hear of references to a lighter grain of 60 mg conversion. The Federal Standards maintain a 64.798 91 mg conversion factor that may be rounded to 65 mg; this is the standard that should be used unless the source specifically states why to use another conversion factor.

Table 9.2 Conversion Factors Format Between the U. S. Customary System and the Metric System (Approximate)

VOLUME

60 μgtt = 1 mL (micro drop)
macrogtt sets varies*
1 tsp = 5 mL
1 Tbsp = 15 mL
1 fl oz = 30 mL
1 cup = 240 mL
1 pt = 480 mL
1 qt = 950 mL
1 gal = 3.8 L
1 L = 1.057 qt

LENGTH		WEIGHT	
1 in	= 2.54 cm	1 gr	= 65 mg
1 ft	= 30.48 cm	1 oz	= 28.35 g
1 yd	= 0.914 m	1 lb	= 0.45 kg
1 mi	= 1.6 km	1 kg	= 2.2 lb
1 m	= 39.37 in	1 g	= 15 gr

*Macrodrop administration sets are variable. Check the product label. The most common macrodrop sets are 10 gtt/mL and 15 gtt/mL.

Note: Some older sources have two conversion factors for grains to milligrams. You may also see or hear of references to a lighter grain of 60 mg conversion. The Federal Standards maintain a 64.798 91 mg conversion factor that may be rounded to 65 mg; this is the standard that should be used unless the source specifically states why to use another conversion factor.

TABLE 9.3 Temperature Conversions

To convert Fahrenheit to Celsius:

$$(°F - 32) \times \frac{5}{9} = °C$$

To convert Celsius to Fahrenheit:

$$\left(°C \times \frac{9}{5}\right) + 32 = °F$$

EXERCISE 9.1 CONVERSIONS BETWEEN SYSTEMS

(Answers may be found in Appendix C.)
(Federal Standards used to calculate answers.)

1. $\frac{1}{4}$ gr = _____ mg

2. 55 lb = _____ kg

3. 45 mL = _____ oz

4. 12 mL = _____ tsp

5. 16.25 mg = _____ gr

6. 12 oz = _____ mL

7. 500 mL = _____ qt

8. 45 mL = _____ oz

9. 2 Tbsp = _____ mL

10. 1 Tbsp = _____ mL

11. $\frac{1}{2}$ gr = _____ mg

12. 1 g = _____ gr

13. gr $\overline{\text{iss}}$ = _____ mg

14. 4 mL = _____ oz

15. 3 oz = _____ mL

16. 180 lb = _____ kg

17. $\frac{1}{6}$ gr = _____ mg

18. 150 lb = _____ kg

19. 260 mg = _____ gr

20. 5.85 g = _____ gr

21. 7 lb = _____ kg

22. 3 oz = _____ mL

23. 11 lb = _____ kg

24. 2 Tbsp = _____ mL

25. 200 lb = _____ kg

26. 0.05 g = _____ gr

27. 0.3 mL = _____ oz

28. $\frac{1}{2}$ gr = _____ mg

29. $1\frac{1}{2}$ gr = _____ mg

30. 30 kg = _____ lb

31. 1000 mL = _____ pt

32. 2000 mL = _____ qt

33. 90 mL = _____ oz

34. 10 mL = _____ cc

35. 2 tsp = _____ mL

36. 2 qt = _____ mL

37. 500 mL = _____ L

38. gr v̄iss = _____ g

39. gr xx = _____ g

40. 220 lb = _____ kg

41. 5 gr = _____ g

42. 88 lb = _____ kg

43. 3 gr = _____ mg

44. 80 kg = _____ lb

45. 50 lb = _____ kg

46. 356 lb = _____ kg

47. 75 gr = _____ g

48. 90 kg = _____ lb

49. 30 mL = _____ Tbsp

50. 80 lb = _____ kg

SECTION THREE

EMERGENCY DRUG DOSAGE CALCULATIONS

This section will address seven of the most common types of emergency drug dosage calculations that will be encountered in the field and in emergency centers, not to mention on exams. Alternative methods of solving these problems have been provided as much as possible. How a problem is solved is not as important as arriving at the correct dose or "drip rate." Continue practicing without a calculator, since most testing institutions will not allow them during exams.

Doctors pour drugs of which they know little, to cure diseases of which they know less, into human beings of whom they know nothing.

—Voltaire—

Find the Ordered Dose

OBJECTIVES

In order to work dosage calculation problems as an emergency health care provider, you should be able to:

1. Recognize the three main components to a simple drug dosage calculation problem.

2. Utilize the key to solving drug dosage calculation problems—*organization.*

3. Solve a basic order word problem using the ratio and proportion method.

4. Solve a basic order word problem by using the formula method.

INTRODUCTION

- *How do I know what the doctor wants?*
- *Which method of solving dosage problems should I use?*

The answers to these questions are simple. What can be difficult is practice! Most students either do not receive enough practice problems or do not choose to practice the problems available to them. The old saying, "Perfect practice makes perfect" holds true. This chapter will explain the problems, provide two methods to solve them, and provide 25 practice problems to help hone your dosage calculation skills.

Measure your mind's height by the shade it casts!
—Elizabeth Barrett Browning—

10.1 FIND THE ORDERED DOSE

In this type of problem, you will be given an order to administer a medication to a patient. There are three components to locate in this type of problem: the doctor's order, the concentration of the drug, and what unit you are about to administer (what you are looking for).

The Doctor's Order

The order should include the amount of medication and the route. The most common routes of administration are endotracheal, intravenous, intramuscular, subcutaneous, sublingual, rectal, or oral. The orders can be verbal, written as standing orders, or hospital nursing orders. Many will be given over portable telephones or radios. Of course, there will always be those orders on the test. Either way, you must be able to pick out *what* the doctor wants to give and by *what route* it is to be administered. The order in the following example is referred to as a **basic order.** It's easy to work with.

Concentration

The second item to identify is the concentration. You will either be given the concentration of a vial, ampule, prefilled syringe, or tablet in a word problem. You may have to choose the correct concentration from what is available in your ambulance, drug box, med-cabinet, or test station. Concentrations can be listed as common fractions, ratio percentages, percentage solutions, or per tablet. The concentration is often worded as what's "on hand."

What Are You Looking For?

It is important to look at the doctor's order and identify the *unit of measurement* that will be administered to the patient, such as milliliters, tablets, and so on. This is the "how much" from your doctor's order. It is usually obvious once the doctor's order has been identified. See if you can find all three components in the following example:

Example: A doctor orders 2 milligrams of Valium™ to be administered I.V. to a patient experiencing seizures. You have a 5-milliliter vial that contains 10 milligrams of Valium™ (10 mg/5 mL). How many milliliters are you going to draw into a syringe and push I.V. into your patient?

The Key

The key to solving dosage calculations is *organization*. Identifying the key components is essential. Developing the habit of organization early will make dosage calculation problems *easy*. This example may seem simple now, but the problems become increasingly difficult. If you develop some simple habits now, the more difficult problems will seem so much easier later. So, before starting any calculation, write down (1) the order, (2) "what's on hand," and (3) what it is you're looking for, as has been done here (the example has been provided, again, for your convenience):

Example: A doctor orders 2 milligrams of Valium™ to be administered I.V. to a patient experiencing seizures. You have a 5-milliliter vial that contains 10 milligrams of Valium™ (10 mg/5 mL). How many milliliters are you going to draw into a syringe and push I.V. into your patient?

Order:	2 mg Valium™, I.V.
On hand:	10 mg/5 mL Valium™
Looking for:	mL

Now that you have the information identified and organized, you may choose one of two methods to solve this problem. They are mathematically similar. Some people just prefer one over the other. Choose the one you are most comfortable with and stick with it.

Ratio and Proportion Method. One way to solve this type of problem is using the ratio and proportion method. For a review of this method see Chapter 3.

1. On the left side of the proportion, put the ratio that is known:

$$10 \text{ mg} : 5 \text{ mL} ::$$

2. On the right side of the proportion, put the ratio that is unknown (usually the ratio composed of the order) and *make sure the units are in the same sequence:*

$$10 \text{ mg} : 5 \text{ mL} :: 2 \text{ mg} : X \text{ mL}$$

3. Now, multiply the extremes. Then, multiply the means:

$$10X = 5 \times 2$$

4. Multiply the right side:

$$10X = 10$$

5. Divide both sides by the number in front of X *and* check to see if the answer's unit matches what you were looking for:

$$X = \textbf{1 mL}$$

Very similar to the ratio and proportion method is cross-multiplication. It simply sets the problem up with common fractions. (See Section 1.1 for a review of cross-multiplication.)

$$\frac{10 \text{ mg}}{5 \text{ mL}} = \frac{2 \text{ mg}}{X \text{ mL}}$$

The math works out exactly the same. Some people just "see" a problem this way.

Formula Method. Some people prefer to use a formula to solve this type of problem. The following formula will be helpful:

$$\text{volume to be administered } (X) = \frac{\text{volume on hand} \times \text{ordered dose}}{\text{concentration (mg, etc.)}}$$

The volume on hand equals the quantity of drug in the container such as milliliters in a vial or premixed syringe from "what's on hand." It could even indicate a single tablet. The concentration is the mass of medication in that volume or tablet from "what's on hand." The ordered dose is what medical control or standing orders dictate.

Example: A doctor orders 2 milligrams of Valium™ to be administered I.V. to a patient experiencing seizures. You have a 5-milliliter vial that contains 10 milligrams of Valium™ 10 mg/5 mL). How many milliliters are you going to draw into a syringe and push I.V. into your patient?

Before you even begin, organize the information:

Order:	2 mg Valium™, I.V.
On hand:	10 mg/5 mL Valium™
Looking for:	mL

1. Fill in the formula.

$$X = \frac{5 \text{ mL} \times 2 \text{ mg}}{10 \text{ mg}}$$

2. Multiply the top. (The mg on top cancels the mg on the bottom. This will leave the unit of mL. Check to see if that is what you are looking for.)

$$X = \frac{10}{10} \text{ mL}$$

3. Reduce the fraction.

$$X = \mathbf{1 \text{ mL}}$$

Both the ratio and proportion method and the formula method can be used with orders involving tablets, pills, I.M., S.Q., or I.V. administration.

Practice Problem. You are caring for a patient with congestive heart failure. The patient is in the tripod position and complaining of difficulty breathing. The patient is using accessory muscles for respirations, and audible heavy crackles are apparent upon auscultation of the chest. As *part* of your standing orders, you are to administer 40 milligrams of Lasix™ I.V. before calling medical control. You have been put in charge of the medication. The vial in the ambulance reads 80 mg/10 mL. How many milliliters do you push?

Answer: 5 mL

EXERCISE 10.1 FIND THE ORDERED DOSE

(Answers may be found in Appendix D.)

Directions: Answer the following drug dosage calculation problems.

1. You are on the scene with a pulseless and apneic patient in ventricular fibrillation. The doctor orders 1 milligram of epinephrine I.V. The medication comes as 0.1 mg/mL. How many milliliters will you give?

2. Medical Control orders 200 milligrams of lidocaine I.V. for your patient in ventricular tachycardia. The prefilled syringe reads "50 mg/mL." How many milliliters will you administer?

3. Your patient meets the criteria for the standing order of 0.5 milligrams of atropine sulfate I.V. It comes supplied in your ambulance as 1 mg/10 mL. How many milliliters will you give?

4. You receive an order in the Emergency Center to administer 100 mEq of sodium bicarbonate I.V. Your prefilled syringe label reads "50 mEq/50 mL." How many milliliters will you administer?

5. A radio order is received from Medical Control to administer 10 milligrams of diazepam (Valium) I.V.P. to your patient experiencing grand mal seizures. Your vial reads "5 mg/mL." How many milliliters will you administer?

6. You are assessing a patient in severe congestive heart failure and Medical Control orders 5 milligrams of morphine sulfate I.V. The prefilled syringe reads "15 mg/mL." How many milliliters will you administer?

7. Your patient is bradycardic and you are ordered to administer 0.6 milligrams of atropine sulfate I.V. The prefilled syringe reads "0.4 mg/mL." How many milliliters will you administer?

8. The patient in the Emergency Center is suffering from congestive heart failure. The doctor orders 80 milligrams of furosemide (Lasix) p.o. The bottle of tablets reads "40 milligrams per tablet." How many tablets will you give?

9. Your patient is a known congestive heart failure patient with very "noisy" lung fields and shortness of breath. Medical control orders 40 milligrams of furosemide (Lasix) I.V. The vial reads "10 mg/mL." How many milliliters will you administer?

10. The patient in the Emergency Center is diagnosed with atrial fibrillation with a rapid ventricular response. The doctor orders 0.25 milligrams of digoxin (Lanoxin) I.V. The vial reads "0.5 mg/mL." What will you give the patient?

11. Your patient is pulseless, apneic, and in asystole. Medical Control orders 0.75 milligrams of epinephrine I.V. Your prefilled syringe reads "1 mg/mL." How many milliliters will you administer?

12. You are on a long transfer with a severe burn patient in a great amount of pain. Meperidine (Demerol) 75 milligrams has been ordered I.M. The prefilled syringe reads "100 mg/mL." How many milliliters will you administer?

13. Your patient is exhibiting paroxysmal supraventricular tachycardia (PSVT). Vagal maneuvers are ineffective and Medical Control orders 6 milligrams adenosine (Adenocard) rapid I.V. The vial reads "3 mg/mL." How many milliliters will you administer?

14. The dose in problem 13 was ineffective. After two minutes, Medical Control orders to increase the dose to 12 milligrams rapid I.V. How many milliliters will you administer now?

15. You arrive in the Emergency Center with the patient from problems 13 and 14. He is still exhibiting PSVT, and the doctor orders you to administer 2.5 milligrams verapamil (Isoptin) slow I.V. The vial reads "5 mg/5 mL." How many milliliters will you administer?

16. A patient's V-Fib. is refractory to lidocaine and defibrillation attempts. Medical Control orders 400 milligrams of Bretylium over one minute I.V. The prefilled syringe reads "50 mg/mL" (10 mL total). How many milliliters will you administer?

17. The bretylium tosylate (Bretylol) is ineffective with the patient from problem 16. Medical Control orders 100 milligrams procainamide to be administered I.V. over five minutes. The vial reads "1 g/10 mL." How many milliliters will you draw up and administer?

18. A patient is exhibiting an agonal arrhythmia. The second dose from the standing orders call for 3 milligrams of epinephrine. The prefilled syringe reads "1 mg/10 mL." How many milliliters will you administer?

19. A patient's Dextro-stix™ is approximately 40 mg/dL, and she is unconscious. Medical Control orders 25 grams of dextrose I.V. bolus. The prefilled syringe reads "0.5 g/mL." How many milliliters will you administer?

20. A patient is suspected of overdosing on heroin. Standing orders call for 2 milligrams of naloxone (Narcan) I.V. The prefilled syringe reads "0.4 mg/mL." How many milliliters will you administer?

21. The patient in the Emergency Center is in hypertensive crisis. The protocol calls for 20 milligrams nifedipine (Procardia) to be squirted out of a pierced capsule into the patient's mouth for sublingual administration. The bottle reads "10 mg/tablet." How many tablets will be used?

22. A patient's blood pressure is dangerously low following a myocardial infarction (M.I). The doctor orders 400 milligrams of dopamine (Intropin) to be added to an I.V. bag. The vial reads "80 mg/mL." How many milliliters will you add to the bag?

23. A patient in mild anaphylaxis needs 75 milligrams diphenhydramine (Benadryl). The prefilled syringe reads "100 mg/5 mL." How many milliliters will you administer?

24. A patient took 30–40 acetaminophen tablets a few minutes ago. The bottle reads 80 milligrams each tablet. Approximately how many milligrams were swallowed?

25. An alcoholic in delirium tremens ("D.T.s") needs 100 milligrams thiamine. You saw the nurse give half of a prefilled syringe that reads "100 mg/mL" (1 mL total). How many milligrams did the nurse give?

26. Your 3-month-old pediatric patient has a high fever. Standing orders call for 40 mg of acetaminophen (Tylenol) to be administered to patients between 0–3 months. You have liquid acetaminophen at a concentration of 160 mg/5 mL available. How many milliliters do you administer?

27. A 24-year-old asthma patient has self-administered three actuations of an albuterol (Proventil) inhaler before your arrival. Each actuation delivers 90 μg of albuterol. How many total micrograms has the patient received?

28. A 50-year-old female patient in cardiac arrest shows V-Fib on the monitor. The V-Fib has been refractory to other treatments and the doctor orders 300 mg slow I.V. of amiodarone (Cordarone). It comes

supplied to ampules of 50 mg/mL (3 mL total). How many milliliters will you administer?

29. After giving the second dose of adenosine to your 38-year-old female in supraventricular tachycardia (SVT), the arrhythmia persists. Standing orders call for the administration of 25 mg of diltiazem (Cardizem) slow I.V. Supplied in your drug box are 5 mL vials with 5 mg/mL. How many milliliters will you administer?

30. A 17-year-old male is experiencing a severe allergic reaction. You are ordered to administer 0.3 mg of 1 : 1000 epinephrine subcutaneously. It comes in ampules of 1 mg/mL. How many milliliters will you administer?

31. A patient with chronic back pain is being prepared for a long transport. Protocols allow for 15 mg ketorolac (Toradol) to be administered I.V. It comes supplied in a 2 mL prefilled syringe labeled 30 mg/mL. How many milliliters will you administer?

32. Over a 15-minute period you have administered three metered-dose sprays of nitroglycerin (Nitrostat) to your 38-year-old patient with chest pain. If each metered dose supplies 0.4 mg nitroglycerin, how many total milligrams have you administered?

33. A patient with profound nausea and vomiting is alert and has taken no alcohol or other sedatives. Standing orders call for 12.5 mg of promethazine (Phenergan) to be administered I.V. It comes supplied in ampules of 25 mg/mL. How many milliliters will you administer?

34. As part of the severe anaphylaxis protocol, you are instructed to give 250 mg methylprednisolone (Solu-Medrol). It comes supplied in 125 mg/2 mL vials. (a) How many milliliters will you administer? (b) How many vials will you use?

35. You are ordered to administer 2 mg of haloperidol (Haldol) to a patient experiencing an acute psychotic episode. The ampule reads "5 mg/mL." How many milliliters will you administer?

36. A patient in hypertensive crisis has orders for labetalol (Normodyne, Trandate) 20 mg slow I.V. It is supplied as 100 mg in 20 mL solvent ampules (5 mg/mL). How many milliliters will you administer?

37. Your patient is a 19-year-old with severe asthma. Terbutaline (Brethine) 0.25 mg subcutaneous is part of the standing orders. It comes supplied in 1 mg/mL ampules. How many milliliters will you administer?

38. As part of the Nontraumatic Chest Pain protocol, you may administer morphine sulfate in 2 mg increments every 5–10 minutes up to a maxi-

mum of 10 mg. The vial reads "10 mg/1 mL." How many milliliters will you administer for your first doses?

39. A patient is in V-Fib and has received his initial defibrillations. Standing orders call for 1 mg epinephrine (Adrenalin) 1:10000 I.V. The prefilled syringe reads "0.1 mg/mL." How many milliliters will you administer?

40. You are asked to put 200 mg of dopamine (Intropin) in a 250 mL I.V. bag. Dopamine comes supplied in 400 mg/5 mL vials. How many milliliters will you put into the bag?

Find the Units Per Kilogram

OBJECTIVES

In order to work dosage calculation problems as an emergency health care provider, you should be able to:

1. Recognize an order based on patient's weight.

2. Utilize the key to solving drug dosage calculation problems—*organization.*

3. Solve an order by patient weight problem using the simple three-step method.

INTRODUCTION

- *This sounds a little complicated. Can I do this?*

Sure you can! Except for one very easy step, everything to solve this problem has already been presented. It's natural for a lot of people to feel nervous when it comes to calculating drug dosages. Read through the three-step method slowly, and you'll find yourself feeling more and more confident with every practice problem you work.

The life is so short, the craft so long to learn.
—Hippocrates—

11.1 FIND THE UNITS PER KILOGRAM

This type of problem adds a new dimension to the problems in Chapter 10. The addition is quite simple. So, if you are able to find the ordered dose, you will have little difficulty with this chapter. Organization is still the key.

The three basic components of a dosage calculation problem—the doctor's order, the concentration (what's "on hand"), and what unit you are to administer—are still the key aspects. The addition is in the doctor's order and the patient's weight. Instead of a basic order (2 milligrams of Valium), the doctor will order a certain number of units (grams, milligrams, etc.) of a drug to be administered based on the patient's weight, almost always in kilograms. This is referred to as an **order based on patient's weight.** Look at the following example:

Example: The doctor orders 5 milligrams per kilogram (5 mg/kg) of bretylium tosylate (Bretylol) I.V. to be administered to your patient. You have premixed syringes with 500 mg/10 mL. Your patient weighs 220 pounds.

    a.   How many milligrams will you administer?
    b.   How many milliliters will you administer?

You can see that the order of 5 milligrams per kilogram of bretylium is a little different. Start by writing down all the key information. In this type of problem, add a patient weight category.

Order:	5 mg/kg bretylium, I.V.
On hand:	500 mg/10 mL bretylium
Looking for:	mL
Pt's weight:	**220 lb**

Look at the order. It is directly tied to the patient's weight. Put another way, the order is saying, "For every kilogram of patient, give 5 milligrams of bretylium." To solve this problem, the order must be converted to a basic order like those in Chapter 10. Since medical orders are going to be in kilograms (metric) and most people know their weight in pounds (customary), it will require converting the patient's weight in pounds to kilograms. Then, it will require converting the order based on patient weight in kilograms to a basic order. Finally, the basic ordered dose can be calculated.

So, there are three steps to this type of problem. First, convert the patient's weight to kilograms. Second, convert the ordered dose based on patient's weight to a basic order. And, third, find the ordered dose. You have done step 1 in Chapter 9. You have performed step 3 in Chapter 10. The only new step is step 2. Always begin with organizing the information:

Example: The doctor orders 5 milligrams per kilogram of bretylium tosylate (Bretylol) I.V. to be administered to your patient. You have premixed syringes 500 mg/10 mL. Your patient weighs 220 pounds.

    a.   How many milligrams will you administer?
    b.   How many milliliters will you administer?

Order:	5 mg/kg bretylium, I.V.
On hand:	500 mg/10 mL bretylium
Looking for:	mL
Pt's weight:	220 lb

Step 1: Convert Pounds to Kilograms

$$220 \text{ lb} \div 2.2 = 100 \text{ kg}$$

or

$$220 \text{ lb} \times 0.45 = 99 \text{ kg}$$

For ease of computation, 99 kg could then be approximated to 100 kg. See Chapter 9 for how to convert pounds to kilograms.

Step 2: Order by Weight to a Basic Order

Step 2 can be calculated by either using a formula or using the ratio and proportion method. The formula method is presented first.

Formula Method. $\quad X = \dfrac{\text{ordered dose} \times \text{weight (kg)}}{1 \text{ kg}}$

1. Set up the formula.

$$X = \frac{5 \text{ mg} \times 100 \text{ kg}}{1 \text{ kg}}$$

kg on top cancels kg on bottom, leaving mg.

2. Work the problem.

$$X = \textbf{500 mg} \text{ of bretylium}$$

This is the basic ordered dose. It answers part (a) of the question. Step 2 can also be performed using the ratio and proportion method.

Ratio and Proportion Method.

$$5 \text{ mg} : 1 \text{ kg} :: X \text{ mg} : 100 \text{ kg}$$

$$X = 5 \times 100$$

$$X = \textbf{500 mg}$$

Either way, this is now a basic order that can be worked with. Draw a line through the order based on patient weight and write in the new basic order of 500 mg over it. This habit will really help keep information organized. Now, the ordered dose must be calculated. This will answer part (b) of the question.

Step 3: Find the Ordered Dose

Since you are already familiar with this step, find the ordered dose using the method you prefer from Chapter 10.

Answer: 10 mL

Now, work the following practice problem.

> **Practice Problem.** You are ordered to give 10 milligrams per kilogram of bretylium tosylate (Bretylol) to your 198-pound patient. You have available premixed syringes with 500 mg/10 mL. How many milliliters will you administer?
>
> Answer: 18 mL

EXERCISE 11.1 FIND THE UNITS PER KILOGRAM

(Answers may be found in Appendix D)

Directions: Answer the following drug dosage calculation problems (round to nearest tenth).

1. Your 150-pound patient is experiencing multifocal premature ventricular contractions (P.V.C.s) and complains of chest pain. Your standing orders state to administer 1 mg/kg of lidocaine. The lidocaine in your ambulance reads "100 mg/5 mL."

   a. How many milligrams will you administer?
   b. How many milliliters will you administer?

2. Your patient from above does not respond to the lidocaine and Medical Control orders 5 mg/kg of bretylium tosylate (Bretylol) I.V. Bretylium is supplied in prefilled syringes containing 500 mg/10 mL.

   a. How many milligrams will you administer?
   b. How many milliliters will you administer?

3. The doctor orders 0.01 mg/kg atropine I.V. for your bradycardic patient who weighs 130 pounds. The atropine in your ambulance reads "1 mg/mL."

   a. How many milligrams will you administer?
   b. How many milliliters will you administer?

4. You are ordered to administer sodium bicarbonate at 1 mEq/kg to a patient who weighs 160 pounds. It is supplied by the Emergency Center's med-cabinet in prefilled syringes that read "50 mEq/50 mL."

   a. How many milligrams will you administer?
   b. How many milliliters will you administer?

5. You have a severely bradycardic 40-pound pediatric patient who does not respond to your initial treatments. You receive an order from Medical Control to administer epinephrine 0.01 mg/kg I.V. Your ampule reads "10 mg/10 mL."

   a. How many milligrams will you administer?
   b. How many milliliters will you administer?

6. A 10-month-old pediatric patient who weighs 13 pounds presents with supraventricular tachycardia (SVT) and requires 0.1 mg/kg of adenosine (Adenocard). The vial reads, "3 mg/mL."

   a. How many milligrams will you administer?
   b. How many milliliters will you administer?

7. The first dose in problem 6 does not convert the supraventricular tachycardia (SVT) in your patient. The second dose is ordered at 0.2 mg/kg.

   a. How many milligrams will you administer?
   b. How many milliliters will you administer?

8. A 26-pound pediatric patient in asystole requires 0.02 mg/kg of atropine sulfate. Atropine comes supplied for pediatrics in 0.5 mg/mL prefilled syringes.

   a. How many milligrams will you administer?
   b. How many milliliters will you administer?

9. A 15-year old newly diagnosed diabetic patient who weighs 100 pounds has taken her insulin and not eaten. Your glucometer shows a blood sugar of 45 mg/dL. The standing orders call for 0.5 g/kg of 50% Dextrose. 50% dextrose comes supplied in 0.5 mg/mL prefilled syringes.

   a. How many milligrams will you administer?
   b. How many milliliters will you administer?

10. A 7-year-old, 45-pound male is in moderate anaphylaxis. You are ordered to administer 2 mg/kg of diphenhydramine (Benadryl). Diphenhydramine comes supplied in prefilled syringes of 50 mg/mL.

    a. How many milligrams will you administer?
    b. How many milliliters will you administer?

11. Your 222-pound patient has converted from V-Fib. His blood pressure is extremely low. Standing orders call for 5 μg/kg of dopamine hydrochloride (Intropin) per minute. How many micrograms per minute is the doctor ordering for this patient?

12. High-dose epinephrine (defined as 0.2 mg/kg by standing orders) is indicated for your patient in cardiac arrest who weighs approximately 180 pounds. You choose a multidose vial of 1:1000 epinephrine that has 30 mg/30 mL.

    a. How many milligrams will you administer?
    b. How many milliliters will you administer?

13. The initial dose of pediatric epinephrine in asystole is 0.1 mg/kg. If your patient weighs 24 pounds and you are instructed to use 1:10000 epinephrine (0.1 mg/mL):

    a. How many milligrams will you administer for your first dose?
    b. How many milliliters will you administer?

14. To sedate your patient for a Rapid Sequence Induction/Intubation (RSI), standing orders call for 0.3 mg/kg of etomidate (Amidate, Hypnomidate). Your patient weighs 260 pounds. If etomidate comes supplied in 20 mL vials at 2 mg/mL:

    a. How many milligrams will you administer?
    b. How many milliliters will you administer?

15. To facilitate intubation of your patient, succinylcholine (Anectine) 1.5 mg/kg is ordered after sedation. The patient weighs 260 pounds. Succinylchloine is supplied in 100 mg/5 mL ampules.

    a. How many milligrams will you administer?
    b. How many milliliters will you administer?
    c. How many ampules must you use to get that dose?

16. After intubation, vecuronium (Norcuron) is indicated to sustain paralysis/skeletal muscle relaxation. A dose of 0.1 mg/kg is ordered I.V. on the above 260-pound patient. It comes supplied in 10 mg/10 mL vials.

    a. How many milligrams will you administer?
    b. How many milliliters will you administer?
    c. How many vials must you use to get that dose?

17. A patient with a history of congestive heart failure is having extreme difficulty breathing and has severely "wet" lung sounds. As part of your therapy for this patient, you are ordered to administer an initial dose of furosemide (Lasix) at 0.5 mg/kg. Your patient weighs 178 pounds. Furosemide is stocked in your ambulance in 2 mL ampules in a concentration of 10 mg/mL.

    a. How many milligrams will you administer?
    b. How many milliliters will you administer?
    c. How many ampules must you use to get that dose?

18. A patient does not convert out of a V-Fib arrhythmia after initial defibrillations and epinephrine. After the next defibrillation, lidocaine 1.5 mg/kg is indicated. The patiend in arrest weighs approximately 167 pounds. If lidocaine comes supplied as 100 mg/5 mL:

    a. How many milligrams will you administer?
    b. How many milliliters will you administer?

19. A pediatric burn patient is in extreme pain enroute to the hospital. You have orders from the burn center to administer 0.1 mg/kg of morphine sulfate I.V. to your 56-pound patient. Morphine comes supplied in 10 mg/mL vials.

    a. How many milligrams will you administer?
    b. How many milliliters will you administer?

20. Your intubated patient has been in asystole/cardiac arrest for an extended period. Sodium bicarbonate at 1 mEq/kg of an 8.4% (50 mEq/50mL) solution is indicated. The patient weighs approximately 110 pounds.

    a. How many milligrams will you administer?
    b. How many milliliters will you administer?

Solutions and Dilutions

OBJECTIVES

In order to work dosage calculation problems as an emergency health care provider, you should be able to:

1. Define and identify a solution.

2. Define and identify a homogeneous solution.

3. Define and identify a solvent.

4. Define and identify a solute.

5. Define and identify a heterogeneous solution.

6. Define and identify an aqueous solution.

7. Define and identify a gaseous solution.

8. Define and identify an alloy.

9. Define concentration.

10. Define and identify a weight/weight percent.

11. Define and identify a volume/volume percent.

12. Define and identify a weight/volume percent.

13. Define and identify a ratio solution.

14. Recognize and solve a weight/volume percent dilution problem.

15. Dilute 50% dextrose to 25% dextrose.

16. Recognize and solve a ratio dilution problem.

INTRODUCTION

- *How can I make 25% dextrose from 50% dextrose?*
- *What happens if I run out of 1:10 000 epinephrine?*

In this chapter, we take a look at solutions and dilutions. Understanding solutions is the basis for understanding diluting a solution. So it might be helpful to review Chapter 4, Percentages.

Even if the job is not particularly enjoyable, enthusiasm
may be high because of the positive benefits it brings.
—Muriel James and John James—

12.1 SOLUTION FUNDAMENTALS

In prehospital and emergency care, percentages describe medications, I.V. fluids, and oxygen concentrations that are administered to patients. These are all administered as solutions. Therefore, it is helpful to understand some of the definitions and expressions associated with solutions.

A **solution** is a homogeneous mixture of two or more substances. A **homogeneous mixture** is uniform throughout. This means that it has the same physical and chemical properties throughout. A saltwater solution is homogeneous. Each time 5 milliliters of a saltwater solution is drawn out, equal parts of salt and water are in each sample. Other examples of solutions or homogeneous mixtures would be the air that we breathe, metal alloys, sodas, and of course, medications. The substance in a solution that is of the greatest quantity is called the **solvent.** The substance dissolved in the solvent is called the **solute.**

A **heterogeneous mixture** has physical and chemical properties that are not uniform throughout. Think for just a moment about a pepperoni pizza.

The parts of a pepperoni pizza are not uniform throughout the whole pizza. Each time an equal slice is cut, different amounts of pepperoni would be on different slices. When this occurs, the mixture is not a solution.

Solutions, in general, may have the solvent in the form of a gas, a liquid, or a solid. Air is an example of a **gaseous solution.** Dry air is composed of 78% nitrogen molecules, 21% oxygen molecules, and 1% argon molecules.

The individual molecules in a gaseous solution are relatively far apart and move independently.

A solution with a solute dissolved in water is called an **aqueous solution.** Body fluids, ocean water, and most injectable medications are all examples of aqueous solutions. The molecules in a liquid solution are closer together than those in a gaseous solution.

Solids can dissolve in one another, too. Many metals dissolve together to form **alloys.** Zinc and copper dissolve together to form brass. Silver and copper form sterling silver. Pills, tablets, and capsules are also examples of **solid solutions.**

Gases, liquids, or solids can be solutes in liquid solvents. Carbon dioxide (gas) is dissolved in carbonated drinks. Acetic acid (liquid) is present in vinegar. Sodium chloride (solid) is dissolved in water to form an I.V. solution. Most emergency medications have liquids or solids dissolved in a liquid solvent, almost always water.

The **concentration** measures the amount of solute in a certain amount of solution or solvent. Concentrated solutions have a large amount of solute for a given amount of solvent. A dilute solution, on the other hand, contains a small amount of solute for a given amount of solvent. There is no definitive demarcation between these descriptions of solutions. In medicine, it is not enough to say, "Hand me some of that concentrated epinephrine" or "Administer some of that dilute lidocaine." A more quantitative measure of concentration is obviously used. To administer therapeutic doses of medicine requires that an accurate method for identifying concentrations be utilized. There are various methods for expressing concentration: molarity, proof, parts per million, percent, and ratio. Of these, percent and ratio are the most common expressions of concentration in emergency health care medications.

There are three ways in which percentage concentration may be expressed:

1. **Weight/weight percent** expresses the number of grams of solute in 100 grams of solution. This means that the *total* weight of both components equals 100 grams.

2. **Volume/volume percent** expresses the number of milliliters of solute in a total volume of 100 mL of solution.

3. **Weight/volume percent** is the most commonly used percentage concentration with emergency medications. It expresses the number of grams of solute in a total volume of 100 mL of solution. When concentration is expressed as a percentage, it is assumed to be weight/volume unless otherwise indicated.

For example, 50% dextrose is a common emergency drug expressed as a weight/volume percentage (see Figure 12.1). This means that there are 50 grams (50 g) of dextrose in every 100 milliliters (100 mL) of the solution.

Ratio Solutions

Another way to express concentration in a solution is by using a ratio. These are not as common as weight/volume percent, but there are still a

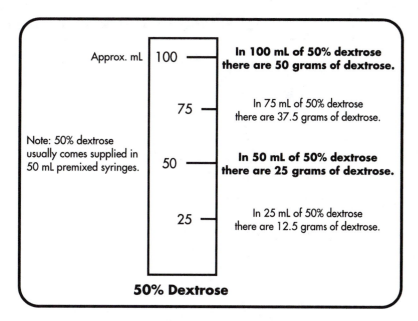

Figure 12.1 Weight/volume percent.

number of medications on ambulances and in emergency centers that use ratios to express concentration. **Ratio solutions** are expressed as 1 gram of a drug in 100 mL, 1000 mL, or 10 000 mL of solvent. Epinephrine is a common drug expressed as a ratio solution. This drug is commonly supplied as 1:1000 and 1:10 000 epinephrine. This is how the ratios will appear and what they mean:

$$1:000 = 1 \text{ g per } 1000 \text{ mL}$$

$$1:10000 = 1 \text{ g per } 10000 \text{ mL}$$

Look at the ratio solutions expressed as fractions:

$$\mathbf{1:1000} = \frac{1 \text{ g}}{1000 \text{ mL}} = \frac{1000 \text{ mg}}{1000 \text{ mL}} = \frac{1 \text{ mg}}{1 \text{ mL}}$$

The 1 milligram per 1 milliliter concentration is the origin of the medical jargon of "one to one epi." Remember that, for proper documentation, the correct ratio solution expression should be 1:1000 or the proper weight/volume percentage of $\frac{1 \text{ mg}}{1 \text{ mL}}$ should be used.

$$\mathbf{1:10000} = \frac{1 \text{ g}}{10000 \text{ mL}} = \frac{1000 \text{ mg}}{10000 \text{ mL}} = \frac{1 \text{ mg}}{10 \text{ mL}}$$

The 1 milligram per 10 milliliter concentration is the origin of the medical jargon of "one to ten epi." Remember that, for proper documentation, the correct ratio solution expression should be 1:10 000 or the proper weight/volume percentage of $\frac{1 \text{ mg}}{10 \text{ mL}}$ should be used.

(Answers may be found in Appendix D.)

Directions: Answer the following questions about percentage and ratio solutions.

1. A mixture that has physical and chemical properties that are uniform throughout is known as a:

    a. heterogeneous mixture
    b. homogeneous mixture
    c. solution
    d. Both b and c are correct

2. A solution with a solute dissolved in a solvent of water is a(an):

    a. heterogeneous mixture
    b. alloy
    c. aqueous solution
    d. simple solution

3. The percent sign (%) means:

    a. "for every hundred"
    b. "for every thousand"
    c. "divided by one hundred thousand"
    d. none of the above

4. Percents are merely fractions with denominators of:

    a. 10
    b. 100
    c. 1000
    d. none of the above

5. The percent that expresses the number of grams of solute in a total volume of 100 mL of solution is a:

    a. weight/weight percent
    b. volume/volume percent
    c. weight/volume percent
    d. any of the above

6. A medication label reads, "2% Lidocaine." This means there are 2 _____ of Lidocaine in every _____ mL of solution.

    a. grams/100
    b. milligrams/100
    c. micrograms/10
    d. none of the above

7. A ratio solution expresses 1 gram of a drug in 100 mL, 1000 mL, or 10000 mL of solvent.

    a. True

    b. False

12.2 DILUTION PROBLEMS

Diluting is the process of adding more solvent to a solution in order to make it less concentrated. Diluting medications, although not all that common, may be necessary in special situations (e.g., pediatric patients or cardiac arrest). The two most common ways to express percent in solutions in emergency medicine is the weight/volume percent and ratio solutions.

Weight/Volume Percent

One type of dilution problem involves diluting a weight/volume percentage. Typically, what is on hand is usually too concentrated to administer to the patient. In emergency medicine, this could be $D_{25}W$ being ordered for a pediatric patient. $D_{50}W$ is usually the concentration most familiar to prehospital and emergency room care providers. Since $D_{50}W$ is twice as concentrated as $D_{25}W$, the dilution is 1 to 1. Look at the following example.

Example: Medical Control orders 1 g/kg of 25% dextrose to be administered to your 22-pound 10-month-old pediatric patient. You only have a prefilled syringe of 50% dextrose in 50 milliliters (25 grams dextrose) and several vials of sterile water. How will you administer this order?

First, find the grams per kilogram the doctor is ordering (see Chapter 11, Find the Units per Kilogram). (Answer: 10 g of 25% dextrose.)

Compare $D_{50}W$ to $D_{25}W$ and make 25% dextrose from what's available. 50% dextrose is twice as concentrated as 25% dextrose. Will it be possible to dilute the 50% dextrose on hand to 25% dextrose? Yes. How can that be accomplished with the standard equipment available in an ambulance or emergency room? If you recall, 50% dextrose comes supplied in 50-milliliter prefilled syringes. Each syringe of 50% dextrose contains 25 grams of dextrose. The 25% dextrose has 12.5 grams of dextrose in 50 milliliters. It is half as concentrated as 50% dextrose (see Figure 12.2).

How to Make 25% Dextrose from 50% Dextrose

1. Take the 50% dextrose and expel half the contents. This will leave 12.5 grams of dextrose in 25 milliliters.

2. Draw 25 milliliters of sterile water or normal saline into the syringe and **mix well.** There are now 12.5 grams of dextrose in 50 milliliters; that is 25% dextrose.

3. Label the syringe.

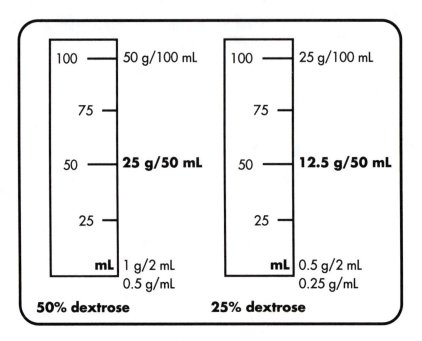

Figure 12.2

4. From the example problem, calculate the ordered dose (see Chapter 10, Find the Ordered Dose).

Answer: 40 mL of 25% dextrose=10 grams.

Practice Problem: Medical Control orders 1 g/kg of 25% dextrose to be administered to your 11-pound, 6-month-old pediatric patient. You only have a prefilled syringe of 50% dextrose in 50 milliliters (25 grams dextrose) and several vials of sterile water.

1. How many total grams of 25% dextrose is the doctor ordering?

2. How can you make $D_{25}W$ from $D_{50}W$?

3. How many milliliters of $D_{25}W$ will you administer?

Answer: (1) 5 g of 25% dextrose. (2) Expel half (25 mL) the $D_{50}W$; draw in 25 mL of sterile water. (3) 20 mL of 25% dextrose.

Ratio Dilutions

The dosage calculation problems involving ratio dilutions typically will ask the student to calculate an ordered dose. Use the steps in Chapter 10, Find the Ordered Dose, to find the answers. Since there is the possibility that a ratio solution may need to be diluted, the following discussion may prove helpful. Look at the following example.

Example: While working a full arrest, the supply of 10-milliliter prefilled syringes of 1 : 10 000 epinephrine is exhausted. There are 10-milliliter syringes, vials of sterile water, and ampules of 1-milliliter 1 : 1000 epinephrine available. The doctor orders 1 milligram of 1 : 10 000 epinephrine I.V. How will this be accomplished?

Understanding ratio solutions makes solving this problem quite easy. Remember that a 1-milliliter ampule of 1:1000 epinephrine contains 1 milligram of drug. The ratio solution of 1 : 1000 means there is 1 gram in 1000 milliliters. This can be converted to the fraction:

$$\frac{1\text{ g}}{1000\text{ mL}}$$

That fraction can then be reduced to how it comes supplied:

$$\frac{1\text{mg}}{1\text{mL}}$$

It is also known that the ratio solution of 1 : 10 000 means there is 1 gram in 10 000 milliliters. This can be converted to the fraction:

$$\frac{1\text{ g}}{10\,000\text{ mL}}$$

That fraction can be reduced to how it comes supplied:

$$\frac{1\text{ mg}}{10\text{ mL}}$$

If there is a solution with 1 milligram in 1 milliliter (1 : 1000) and a solution with 1 milligram in 10 milliliter (1 : 10 000) is needed, all that will be necessary is to draw up the 1 milliliter of 1 : 1000 in a 10-milliliter syringe and then draw in 9 milliliters of sterile water to achieve the 1 : 10 000 concentration. The syringe should be turned upside down several times to ensure adequate mixing.

Other types of ratio problems can be easily solved using either the formula or ratio and proportion method from Chapter 10.

EXERCISE 12.2 SOLUTIONS AND DILUTIONS

(Answers may be found in Appendix D.)

1. Medical Control orders 0.5 g/kg of 25% dextrose to be administered to your 13-pound pediatric patient. You only have a prefilled syringe of 50% dextrose in 50 milliliters (25 grams of dextrose) and vials of sterile water.

    a. How many *total* grams of $D_{25}W$ is the doctor ordering?
    b. How can 25% dextrose be made out of the 50% dextrose available?
    c. How many milliliters of 25% dextrose will be administered to the patient?

2. After first line drugs in a pediatric cardiac arrest, your standing orders call for you to administer 1 g/kg of 25% dextrose. The mother states the infant weighs 9 pounds. Your dextrose is supplied as $D_{50}W$ in 50 milliliters in prefilled syringes. You also have vials of sterile water.

    a. How many *total* grams of $D_{25}W$ is the doctor ordering?

    b. How can 25% dextrose be made out of the 50% dextrose available?

    c. How many milliliters of 25% dextrose will be administered to the patient?

3. The recommended pediatric dose of epinephrine $1:10000$ is 0.1 mL/kg. Based only on the information in this problem, what is the recommended *milligrams per kilogram* pediatric dose of $1:10000$ epinephrine?

4. You have just administered 0.5 mL of a $1:1000$ epinephrine solution to a patient in anaphylaxis. How many milligrams did you administer?

5. A 2 year old has converted from cardiac arrest. You are ordered to administer 1 g/kg of a $D_{25}W$ solution, monitor, and transport. With your $D_{50}W$ and sterile water, how many milliliters of $D_{25}W$ are you going to administer to your 35-pound patient?

6. You have 1 milligram of epinephrine in 10 milliliters. How would this be expressed in a ratio dilution?

7. You are ordered to give 1 milligram of $1:10000$ epinephrine. Your med-drawer is out of $1:10000$. However, you have several 1-milliliter vials of $1:1000$ epinephrine, syringes, and sterile water. How many milliliters of sterile water will you add to what you draw from one vial of $1:1000$ to arrive at the $1:10000$ concentration for the second dose?

8. A vial of epinephrine reads "1 mg/1 mL." What is the ratio dilution?

9. Postarrest of a $4\frac{1}{2}$-pound neonate, you are ordered to push 1 g/kg of $D_{10}W$. You only have $D_{50}W$ to dilute with sterile water.

    a. How many *total* grams of $D_{10}W$ is the doctor ordering?

    b. How can 10% dextrose be made out of the 50% dextrose available?

    c. How many milliliters of 10% dextrose will be administered to the patient?

Find the Concentration

OBJECTIVES

In order to work dosage calculation problems as an emergency health care provider, you should be able to:

1. Recognize the two basic types of concentration problems.

2. Find the concentration of a solution into which a drug has been added using either the formula or ratio and proportion methods.

3. Find the amount of solute in a weight/volume percent solution using either the formula or ratio and proportion methods.

INTRODUCTION

- *How do I find the concentration if a drug has been added to a solution?*
- *How do I find the amount of solute in a solution?*

There are two types of concentration problems that you will encounter as an emergency care provider. The first is a step to solving I.V. drip problems. The second tests your knowledge of the solutions you work with. Two methods, the formula and the ratio and proportion method, are provided to help you solve them.

Excellence is never an accident.
—A Father's Book of Wisdom—

13.1 FIND THE CONCENTRATION

In most facilities and E.M.S. systems, the pharmacy or drug manufacturer prepares solutions for I.V. use. However, in small hospitals, rural E.M.S. systems, and other settings (such as testing sites), you will be required to measure, prepare, and administer these solutions. There are usually two types of concentration problems encountered in emergency care and testing. One is simply finding the concentration, and the other asks for the amount of solute in a certain amount of a weight/volume percentage.

Concentration

The first type of problem is used to find out the concentration of a particular premixed I.V. solution (or syringe or vial, etc.). It is also used as a step in solving or checking other problems. It is important to know the answer to the question, "What do they mean by *concentration?*" The usual answer is how many grams, milligrams, or micrograms of a drug are contained per one milliliter of a given solution. As was explained in the previous chapter, there are certainly many other ways to express concentration. When emergency care workers are referring to an I.V.'s concentration, they usually mean a "per milliliter" concentration.

This is the key to solving I.V. drip problems easily (Chapter 14). You should be able to easily find a "per milliliter" concentration. There is a standard formula that is used to express concentration. Once it is set up, it is simply a matter of reducing the fraction to a denominator of 1.

Formula Method.

$$X = \frac{\text{solute (grams or milligrams of drug)}}{\text{solvent (liters or milliliters of volume)}}$$

Example: One gram of lidocaine has been added to a 250-milliliter bag of D_5W. What is the concentration?

1. Set up the formula:

$$X = \frac{1 \text{ g lidocaine}}{250 \text{ mL } D_5W}$$

2. Convert grams to milligrams (lidocaine is ordered in milligrams):

$$X = \frac{1000 \text{ mg lidocaine}}{250 \text{ mL } D_5W}$$

3. Reduce the fraction to a denominator of 1 by dividing both the numerator and denominator by the denominator:

$$X = \frac{1000 \text{ mg lidocaine}}{250 \text{ mL D}_5\text{W}} \div \frac{250}{250} = \frac{4 \text{ mg}}{1 \text{ mL}}$$

$$X = \frac{4 \text{ mg lidocaine}}{1 \text{ mL D}_5\text{W}}$$

or

$$X = \textbf{4 mg lidocaine/mL D}_5\textbf{W}$$

This can be expressed verbally as "The concentration is 4 milligrams per milliliter" or "4 to 1." This is the "per milliliter" concentration.

Ratio and Proportion. This type of problem can also be solved using the ratio and proportion method. The known concentration is placed on the left and the unknown concentration (per one milliliter) on the right:

$$1000 \text{ mg} : 250 \text{ mL} :: X \text{ mg} : 1 \text{ mL}$$

$$250 \, X = 1000$$

$$X = \frac{1000}{250}$$

$$X = 4 \text{ mg}$$

X is to be placed in the ratio above: $4 \text{ mg} : 1 \text{ mL}$ or $\frac{4 \text{ mg}}{1 \text{ mL}}$.

> **Practice Problem:** A doctor gives you an order to mix 400 milligrams of dopamine into a 250-milliliter bag of D_5W. What will your concentration be? (Dopamine is ordered in micrograms.)
>
>
>
> Answer: Concentration = 1600 μg/mL

Amount of Solute

The second type of concentration problem is seen more often on tests. It is searching for the amount of solute in a weight/volume percent solution. Here are a couple of examples of how this type of problem could be worded:

Example: You have a 250-milliliter bag of D_5W. How many grams of dextrose are in the bag?

Remember that D_5W is expressing the weight/volume percent of 5% dextrose in water (see Chapter 12, Solutions and Dilutions). That means that there are 5 grams of dextrose in 100 milliliters of solution. The basis to solve this problem is now available.

HINT: If the problem asks for answers in milligrams, the grams will need to be converted to milligrams to find the correct answer.

Formula Method. A formula or the ratio and proportion method may be used to solve the example.

$$\text{percent of solution} \times \text{volume of solution} = \text{\# of grams}$$

This example is solved by filling in the formula and working the problem:

$$5\% \text{ or } \frac{5\,g}{100\,mL} \times 250\,mL = \textbf{12.5 g}$$

Ratio and Proportion. This problem could also be worked using either the ratio and proportion or cross-multiplication methods:

$$5\,g : 100\,mL :: X\,g : 250\,mL \qquad \frac{5\,g}{100\,mL} = \frac{X\,g}{250\,mL}$$

$$100\,X = 5 \times 250$$

$$100\,X = 1250$$

$$X = \frac{1250}{100}$$

$$X = \textbf{12.5 g}$$

These same types of problems can be twisted around. What if the number of grams to be administered and the percent were given and the amount to be infused was the unknown? Look at the following example:

Example: The doctor orders 12.5 grams of 5% dextrose to be infused. How many milliliters will be infused?

Again, a formula, the ratio and proportion method, or cross-multiplication may be used to solve this type of problem.

Formula Method. Here is the formula to use in this situation:

$$\text{volume} = \frac{\text{amount ordered (grams)}}{\text{percent}}$$

The example is solved by filling in the formula and working the problem:

$$\text{volume} = \frac{12.5\,g}{5\%}$$

or mathematically the same:

$$\text{volume} = 12.5\,g \div \frac{5\,g}{100\,mL}$$

Either way you work it,

$$\text{volume} = 250\,mL$$

Ratio and Proportion. This problem could also be worked using the ratio and proportion method.

$$5\,g : 100\,mL :: 12.5\,g : X\,mL$$

$$5\,X = 1250$$

$$X = \frac{1250}{5}$$

$$X = 250\,mL$$

(Answers may be found in Appendix D.)

Directions: Answer the following drug dosage calculation problems.

1. The doctor orders 200 milligrams of dopamine to be added to a 250-milliliter bag of D_5W. What is the "per milliliter" concentration in the bag?

2. How many grams of sodium chloride are in a 1000-milliliter bag of 0.9% normal saline?

3. The doctor orders 0.5 grams of aminophylline to be placed in a 100-milliliter bag of D_5W for an I.V. piggyback. What is the "per milliliter" concentration?

4. You are ordered to administer 500 milligrams of a 10% solution of calcium chloride. How many milliliters will you administer?

5. You are ordered to administer an isoproterenol (Isuprel) drip. The doctor orders 2 milligrams to be placed into a 500-milliliter bag of D_5W. What is the concentration?

6. There is a prefilled syringe of 1% lidocaine in your ambulance. It contains 5 milliliters. How many milligrams does it contain?

7. There is also a prefilled syringe of 2% lidocaine in your ambulance. It also contains 5 mL. How many milligrams does it contain?

8. You are ordered to administer a lidocaine drip. The doctor orders 1 gram to be placed into a 250-milliliter bag of D_5W. What is the "per milliliter" concentration?

9. How many grams of dextrose are in a 500-milliliter bag of D_5W?

10. You have a prefilled syringe of lidocaine that reads "100 mg/5 mL." What is the per milliliter concentration?

11. How many grams of sodium chloride are in a 250-milliliter bag of 0.9% normal saline?

12. Standing orders tell you to add 2 grams of lidocaine into a 500-milliliter bag of D_5W. What is the concentration?

13. The label on a vial of furosemide reads 20 mg/2 mL. What is the concentration?

14. The Valium™ vial in your cardiac kit reads "10 mg/2 mL." What is the concentration in the vial?

15. You are reading a label on an 250-milliliter I.V. bag. It states that 400 mg of dopamine were added to it approximately 20 minutes ago. The bag now has 150 mL left in it. What is the "per milliliter" concentration in the bag now?

16. Another patient's bag reads that 1 milligram of epinephrine has been added to his 250-milliliter bag of D_5W. It has been over an hour and there is only 200 milliliter left in the bag. What is the per milliliter concentration of the bag now?

17. The doctor orders you to administer 75 milligrams of 2% lidocaine to your patient experiencing premature ventricular contractions (P.V.C.s) and chest pain. How many milliliters will you administer?

18. Your patient has accidentally overdosed on Cardizem™. The doctor orders 300 milligrams of a 10% solution of calcium chloride I.V. How many milliliters will you administer?

19. 200 milligrams of dopamine have been added to a 250-milliliter bag of normal saline. What is the per milliliter concentration in the bag?

20. The label on a 100-milliliter bag hanging in the ICU reads "1 mg epinephrine added." What is the per milliliter concentration?

Calculate an I.V. Drip Rate

OBJECTIVES

In order to work dosage calculation problems as an emergency health care provider, you should be able to:

1. Recognize an I.V. drip problem.

2. Organize the information from an I.V. drip problem.

3. Recognize and be familiar with the dimensional analysis method of solving I.V. drip problems.

4. Solve an I.V. drip problem using either the dimensional analysis or rule of fours method.

INTRODUCTION

- *How is an I.V. drip calculated?*
- *I've been shown some pretty difficult ways to solve I.V. drip problems. Isn't there an easier way?*

There is an easy way to solve I.V. drip problems. This chapter examines the traditional dimensional analysis method and an easier rule of fours method to calculate I.V. drip problems. In order to use the rule of fours method, you must have mastered how to find the per milliliter concentration in the previous chapter. You choose the method you prefer. It doesn't matter which method you use, as long as you get the correct answer!

Words are, of course, the most powerful drug
used by mankind.
—Rudyard Kipling—

14.1 CALCULATE AN I.V. DRIP RATE

Calculating an I.V. drip has been a quandary for many emergency care providers. Just ask any paramedic, nurse, or doctor to set up an I.V. drip without calculators, references, electric I.V. pumps, or computerized devices, and you will hear all kinds of moans and excuses. But that is exactly what you will be expected to do at test stations all over the country. Being adequately prepared will greatly diminish any anxieties. There are basically two ways to perform this calculation. One is the "hard" way, and the other is the "easy" way. Whichever method you prefer, information organization is still the *key* to solving I.V. drip rate problems. But let's first look at just what an I.V. drip is all about.

I.V. Drip

Sometimes you will be ordered to administer a certain number of milligrams, micrograms, and so on of a medication per minute to a patient through an I.V. This is called an "I.V. drip" because it involves calculating the number of drops that "drip" and are delivered intravenously each minute to deliver the amount of drug the doctor is ordering. This involves drawing medication from a vial or ampule into a syringe or picking a premixed syringe and mixing it into an I.V. bag. Then, you will be required to set a drip rate based upon the doctor's order and the administration set that is available. The final solution is going to usually be the number of drops (gtt) that should fall each minute.

There are many variables in this type of calculation: the order from Medical Control may change, the vial's concentration may vary, the size of the I.V. bag can change, and even though the administration set is usually a 60 gtt/mL set, it too may vary. It is important to develop a system that works for you. First, see the math in what most people call "the hard way." Then, when you understand the algebra behind the problem, we'll learn a very easy and logical method for solving this type of problem.

Formula Method (a.k.a. Dimensional Analysis)

Those of you who have a chemistry or algebra background will not only appreciate this method, you will probably prefer it. It very systematically and mathematically calculates the I.V. drip rate. If you don't particularly like math or chemistry, you probably won't like this method. You *do* still need to review it, though. This method will show you how a drip rate is calculated and answer a lot of questions that may arise later if you do not at least review this method. *Organization* of the material is the key to success. Look at the following example:

Example: A doctor orders 2 milligrams of lidocaine per minute to be administered to a patient who was experiencing an arrhythmia. You have a vial that contains 1 gram of lidocaine in 5 milliliters. Your ambulance carries only 250-milliliter bags of D₅W. Your administration set is a microdrip set (60 gtt/mL). At how many drops per minute will you adjust your administration set to drip?

Before starting any calculations, organize the information just as you were doing in Chapter 10, Find the Ordered Dose. There are a couple of new categories in this type of problem.

Order:	2 mg lidocaine/min I.V.
On hand:	1 g lidocaine/5 mL
Bag:	**250 mL D₅W**
Adm. set:	**60 gtt/mL**
Looking for:	gtt/min

Formula (a.k.a. Dimensional Analysis)

$$X = \frac{\text{I. V. bag volume (mL)}}{\text{Drug in bag}} \times \frac{\text{mg ordered}}{1 \text{ min}} \times \frac{\text{adm. set (gtt)}}{1 \text{ mL}}$$

1. Fill in the formula.

$$X = \frac{250 \text{ mL}}{1 \text{ g}} \times \frac{2 \text{ mg}}{1 \text{ min}} \times \frac{60 \text{ gtt}}{1 \text{ mL}}$$

NOTE: The 5 milliliters in the vial on hand is *not* figured into the equation.

2. Convert the grams in the bag to milligrams (since the order is in milligrams).

$$X = \frac{250 \text{ mL}}{\mathbf{1000 \text{ mg}}} \times \frac{2 \text{ mg}}{1 \text{ min}} \times \frac{60 \text{ gtt}}{1 \text{ mL}}$$

3. Cancel out any units and zeros (Does it leave the units that you are looking for?).

$$X = \frac{25}{10} \times \frac{2}{1 \text{ min}} \times \frac{6 \text{ gtt}}{1}$$

4. Now multiply.

$$X = \frac{300 \text{ gtt}}{10 \text{ min}}$$

5. Reduce the fraction.

$$X = \frac{30 \text{ gtt}}{1 \text{ min}}$$

or

30 gtt/min

You can now set your drip rate on the I.V. administration set. Remember, in most ambulances and test centers, an electric or computerized I.V. pump will not be available, and you will have to set the rate by hand.

"Rule of Fours" Method (a.k.a. The Clock Method)

This method is called "the rule of fours" because it is based on multiples of the number four. This is what a lot of people call the "easy" way. That's because they find it far simpler than the formula method or dimensional analysis. It requires the memorization of a process, not a formula, and requires only simple logic and very little mathematical calculation. Look at the same example problem from before:

Example: A doctor orders 2 milligrams of lidocaine per minute to be administered to a patient who was experiencing an arrhythmia. You have a vial that contains 1 gram of lidocaine in 5 milliliters. Your ambulance carries only 250-milliliter bags of D_5W. Your administration set is a microdrip set (60 gtt/mL). At how many drops per minute will you adjust your administration set to drip?

We begin by organizing the information from the problem similar to how it has been done in previous examples. However, this time we add a new category: the concentration of the I.V. solution (1 g into 250 mL). This is the key in the rule of fours method. For a review of this process see Chapter 13, Find the Concentration.

Order:	2 mg lidocaine/min I.V.
On Hand:	1 g lidocaine/5 mL
Bag:	250 mL D_5W
Conc.:	**4 mg/mL**
Adm. set:	60 gtt/mL
Looking for:	gtt/min

There are three easy steps to the rule of fours method:

1. **Compare.** Now that the information is organized, a logical comparison can be made between the concentration and the administration set. Looking at the concentration we could say that in every 1 milliliter there is 4 milligrams of lidocaine. We could also say that there are 60 drops in each milliliter. Therefore, in every 60 drops there are 4 milligrams. Look at this relationship:

$$4 \text{ mg} = 1 \text{ mL}$$

and

$$60 \text{ gtt} = 1 \text{ mL}$$

therefore,

$$4 \text{ mg} = 60 \text{ gtt}$$

2. **Set up.** Set up the rule of fours clock based on step 1. Drops go on the inside of the clock and milligrams go on the outside. The relationship be-

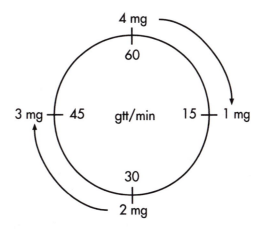

tween the 4 mg and the 60 gtt becomes the 12 o'clock position. Halfway around the clock is the logical half of that relationship. So 30 gtt equals 2 mg and so on around the clock.

3. **Look.** Look at the doctor's order and compare it to the "clock." Find the drops per minute that corresponds to the milligram per minute order. This is the rate at which the administration set is to drip.

$$X = 30 \text{ gtt/min}$$

Different "clocks" can be set up depending upon the concentration in the I.V. bag and/or the administration set available. These parameters can change. The process of setting up the "clock" will be the same and work every time. Work the following practice problem using the method you prefer. See Appendix H for examples of other "clocks."

> **Practice Problem.** The doctor orders 400 micrograms of dopamine per minute (400 μg/min) to be administered by I.V. You have a vial that contains 200 milligrams of dopamine in 10 milliliters (200 mg/ 10 mL). Your ambulance carries only 250-milliliter (250 mL) bags of D$_5$W, and you choose a microdrip administration set (60 gtt/mL). At how many drops per minute will you adjust your administration set to drip?

> Answer: 30 gtt/min

EXERCISE 14.1 CALCULATE AN I.V. DRIP

(Answers may be found in Appendix D.)

1. You are ordered to administer an isoproterenol (Isuprel) drip at 4 μg/min. You are ordered to place 1 milligram into a 250-milliliter bag of D$_5$W. At what rate will you set your microdrip (60 gtt/mL) administration set?

2. Now calculate problem 1 using a macrodrip administration set (10 gtt/ mL).

3. You are ordered to administer lidocaine in an I.V. drip at 2 mg/min. You have 1 gram of lidocaine to add to a 250-milliliter bag. Using a microdrip administration set (60 gtt/mL), at what rate will you set your administration set to drip?

4. Now calculate problem 3 using a macrodrip (10 gtt/mL) administration set.

5. Your patient's blood pressure is critically low following conversion from ventricular fibrillation. Medical Control orders you to mix 400 milligrams of dopamine into a 250-milliliter bag of D_5W and infuse it at 800 μg/min. With your microdrip administration set (60 gtt/mL), at what rate will you infuse the solution?

6. You are ordered to initiate a bretylium tosylate (Bretylol) drip following conversion of multifocal premature ventricular contractions (PVCs). The order is for 1 mg/min. You have 1 g of bretylium, a 250-milliliter bag of D_5W, and a microdrip (60 gtt/mL) administration set. What is the drip rate?

7. In problem 6, what is the drip rate if you only have a macrodrip (15 gtt/mL) administration set?

8. You receive an order to start a dopamine drip at 600 μg/min. You place 200 milligrams of dopamine into a 250-milliliter bag of D_5W. Using a microdrip set (60 gtt/mL), at what rate will you set your administration set?

9. In problem 8, what is the drip rate if you place 400 milligrams of dopamine in a 500-milliliter bag of D_5W? You still have a microdrip set.

10. You are ordered to administer dopamine by mixing 200 milligrams of dopamine into a 500-milliliter bag of D_5W. The order is for 800 μg/min. Using a microdrip set (60 gtt/mL), at what rate will you set your administration set?

11. In problem 10, what is the drip rate if you only have a macrodrip (15 gtt/ mL) administration set?

12. The doctor orders a starting dose of 2 μg/min of epinephrine. Your assistant has mixed 1 mg of epinephrine into a 250-milliliter bag of normal saline. Using a microdrip set, at what rate will you set your administration set?

13. You are ordered to administer an isoproterenol (Isuprel) drip at 4 μg/min. You are ordered to place 2 milligrams into a 500-milliliter bag

of D_5W. At what rate will you set your microdrip (60 gtt/mL) administration set?

14. Now calculate problem 13 using a macrodrip administration set (10 gtt/ mL).

15. You are ordered to administer lidocaine in an I.V. drip at 2 mg/min. You have 2 grams of lidocaine to add to a 500-milliliter bag. Using a microdrip administration set (60 gtt/mL), at what rate will you set your administration set to drip?

16. Now calculate problem 15 using a macrodrip (10 gtt/mL) administration set.

17. Your patient's blood pressure is critically low following conversion from ventricular fibrillation. Medical Control orders you to mix 200 milligrams of dopamine into a 250-milliliter bag of D_5W and infuse it at 400 μg/min. With your microdrip administration set (60 gtt/mL), at what rate will you infuse the solution?

18. Now calculate problem 17 using 400 milligrams of dopamine.

19. You receive an order to start a dopamine drip at 600 μg/min. You place 800 milligrams of dopamine into a 500-milliliter bag of D_5W. Using a microdrip set (60 gtt/mL), at what rate will you set your administration set?

20. In problem 19, what is the drip rate if you only have a macrodrip (15 gtt/ mL) administration set?

21. While on the scene of a cardiac arrest conversion your supervisor tells you to set up an epinephrine drip. You have one ampule of 1:1000 epinephrine (1 mg/mL) to be placed in a 100 mL I.V. bag. You are instructed to start the drip at 5 μg/min. At what rate will you set the microdrip administration set?

22. You are ordered to place 150 mg of amiodarone (Cordarone) into a 100 mL bag with a macrodrip (10 gtt/mL) administration set and run it at 15 mg/min. At what rate will you set the administration set?

Calculate an I.V. Drip Based on Patient Weight

OBJECTIVES

In order to work dosage calculation problems as an emergency health care provider, you should be able to:

1. Recognize an I.V. drip problem based on patient weight.

2. Organize the information from an I.V. drip problem based on patient weight.

3. Solve an I.V. drip problem based on patient weight using either the dimensional analysis or rule of fours method.

INTRODUCTION

- *How is this different from the previous chapter?*
- *Is this as easy as the rule of fours method?*

This chapter takes what you were doing in the previous chapter just one step further. It adds the dimension of patient weight. It really is quite simple.

Education makes us what we are.
—C.A. Helvétius—

15.1 CALCULATE AN I.V. DRIP BASED ON PATIENT WEIGHT

I.V. drip medication orders can be based on patient weight just as basic orders can. Armed with the knowledge from Chapter 11, Find the Units Per Kilogram, and Chapter 14 on I.V. drips, you already know how to calculate this type of problem. Look at the following example:

> **Example/Practice Problem:** An order is received to administer 10 micrograms per kilogram per minute (10 μg/kg/min) of dopamine I.V. You have a vial that contains 200 milligrams of dopamine in 10 milliliters (200 mg/10 mL). You also have 250-milliliter (250 mL) bags of D$_5$W with a microdrip administration set. Your patient weighs 176 pounds. At how many drops per minute will you adjust your administration set to drip?

Organize the material as before. This time the category of patient weight is added.

Order:	10 μg/kg/min $\rightarrow$ 800 μg/min
On Hand:	200 mg dopamine/10 mL
Bag:	250 mL D$_5$W
Adm. set:	60 gtt/mL
Pt.'s weight:	**176 lb $\rightarrow$ 80 kg**
Looking for:	gtt/min

1. Convert the patient's weight to kilograms and the doctor's order from micrograms per kilogram per minute to micrograms per minute as shown above with the arrows.

2. You now have the ordered dose. Solve the drip rate as you did in Chapter 14.

Answer: 60 gtt/min

EXERCISE 15.1 I.V. DRIP BASED ON PATIENT WEIGHT

(Answers may be found in Appendix D.)

1. An order is received to administer dopamine to a 176-pound patient by mixing 200 milligrams of dopamine into a 250-milliliter bag of D$_5$W. Dopamine is supplied in ampules containing 200 mg/4 mL. The order is to deliver the dopamine at 5 μg/kg/min. At how many drops per minute will you adjust your microdrip administration set to drip?

2. You have just received orders to initiate an epinephrine drip on your 22-pound pediatric patient. The order is to mix 1 milligram of epinephrine into a 250-milliliter bag of D$_5$W and run at 0.1 μg/kg/min. Using a

microdrip administration set, at how many drops per minute will the infusion run?

3. In problem 2, what would the drip rate be if the doctor doubled the dose to 0.2 μg/kg/min?

4. Your 132-pound cardiac patient is in cardiogenic shock. The doctor orders a dopamine drip to be initiated at 10 μg/kg/min. Your partner has just placed 400 milligrams of dopamine hydrochloride (Intropin) into a 500-milliliter bag of D_5W. At how many drops per minute will you adjust your microdrip administration set to drip?

5. You are transporting a 66-pound pediatric patient with a congenital heart defect. The doctor initially orders 20 μg/kg/min of lidocaine to be infused I.V. The nurse hands you a 250-milliliter bag of D_5W that she has labeled "200 milligrams lidocaine added." At how many drops per minute will you adjust your microdrip administration set to drip?

6. The patient in problem 5 does not significantly improve. You are told to increase the current infusion to 40 μg/kg/min. Now what will your infusion rate be?

7. You are completing your report after delivering a patient to the emergency room, and you notice that the dopamine dose ordered by medical control is missing. To avoid any possible reprimands, you decide to determine the ordered dose based on the information available. The patient weighs 176 pounds, and the I.V. infusion is flowing through a microdrip administration set at 30 gtt/min. The label on the 500-milliliter bag of D_5W reads "800 milligrams of dopamine added." What was the original dose per kilogram per minute ordered?

8. You are in the same situation as you were in problem 7. The patient weighs 220 pounds. The infusion set is a microdrip administration set. It is flowing at 30 gtt/min. The label on the 250-milliliter bag of D_5W reads "200 milligrams of dopamine added." What was the original dose per kilogram per minute ordered?

9. Your cardiac patient is exhibiting signs and symptoms of cardiogenic shock. Medical Control orders a dopamine infusion at 3 μg/kg/min. The patient's wife states that her husband weighs about 150 pounds. The vial of dopamine is labeled 200 mg/5 mL. You have a 250-milliliter bag of D_5W. At how many drops per minute will you adjust your microdrip administration set to drip?

10. You are setting up an isoproterenol (Isuprel) drip on your 75-pound pediatric patient suffering from refractory bronchospasm. The doctor has ordered 0.1 μg/kg/min. The vial label reads "1 mg/5 mL." You have a 250-milliliter bag of D_5W with a microdrip administration set. At how many drops per minute will you adjust your microdrip administration set to drip?

Milliliters Per Hour to Drops Per Minute

OBJECTIVES

In order to work dosage calculation problems as an emergency health care provider, you should be able to:

1. Recognize an I.V. order of milliliters per hour that needs to be converted to drops per minute.

2. Fill the information from the problem into the formula.

3. Solve an I.V. order of milliliters per hour that needs to be converted to drops per minute.

INTRODUCTION

- *How do I convert milliliters per hour to drops per minute?*

This chapter takes a look at the conversion of a doctor's order for an I.V. to run in over a certain period of time to drops per minute. A simple conversion formula is all you need.

*The best way to convince a fool that he is wrong is to let
him have his own way.*
—Josh Billings (Henry Wheeler Shaw)—

16.1 MILLILITERS PER HOUR TO DROPS PER MINUTE

Sometimes doctors will order I.V.s to run in *milliliters per hour*. The problem with this type of order is that paramedics, nurses, and other health care professionals need to set I.V. administration sets in *drops per minute*. This is seen more frequently in the emergency center, but it occurs in the field as well. As we have seen in previous chapters, there is a relationship between milliliters and the administration set's drops per minute. There is a simple formula that will help with this type of conversion problem. Look at the following formula and example.

Formula

$$X = \frac{\text{order (mL)}}{\text{order (time)}} \times \frac{\text{adm. set (gtt)}}{1 \text{ mL}}$$

Example: The doctor orders you to start an I.V. of normal saline *to run at* (t.r.a.) 100 milliliters per hour (100 mL/hr). You have a macrodrip set that delivers 15 drops per one milliliter (15 gtt/mL). At how many drops per minute will you set your administration set to drip?

1. When setting up the formula, convert the "hours" in the order into minutes:

$$X = \frac{100 \text{ mL}}{60 \text{ min}} \times \frac{15 \text{ gtt}}{1 \text{ mL}}$$

2. The milliliters now cancel out, leaving the drops per minute (gtt/min) we are looking for. Also, cancel out any zeros.

$$X = \frac{10}{6 \text{ min}} \times \frac{15 \text{ gtt}}{1}$$

3. Now multiply.

$$X = \frac{150 \text{ gtt}}{6 \text{ min}}$$

4. Reduce the fraction.

$$X = \frac{25 \text{ gtt}}{1 \text{ min}}$$

or

25 gtt/min

Practice Problem. The doctor orders you to start an I.V. of normal saline to run at 100 milliliters per hour (100 mL/hr). You have a microdrip set that delivers 60 drops per one milliliter (60 gtt/mL). At how many drops per minute will you set your administration set to drip?

Answer: 100 gtt/min

You have probably already noticed that when a microdrip administration set (60 gtt/mL) is used, the order of milliliters per hour will equal the drops per minute. No calculations are necessary.

This type of problem can be presented in a slightly different way. What if a doctor wants a solution to run in over a certain period of time, like over an eight-hour shift? Look at the following example.

Example: An order is received to administer 500 mL of D$_5$W to run in over five hours. Using a microdrip administration set, at how many drops per minute will you set your administration set to drip?

The formula from the previous example will work just as well with this type of problem.

1. Set up using the formula.

$$X = \frac{500 \text{ mL}}{300 \text{ min}} \times \frac{60 \text{ gtt}}{1 \text{ mL}}$$

2. The milliliters cancel as before. Also, any zeros may be canceled out. Reduce the fraction as necessary.

$$X = \frac{5}{3 \text{ min}} \times \frac{60 \text{ gtt}}{1}$$

3. Multiply.

$$X = \frac{300 \text{ gtt}}{3 \text{ min}}$$

4. Reduce.

$$X = \frac{100 \text{ gtt}}{1 \text{ min}}$$

or

$$100 \text{ gtt/min}$$

This formula can be used no matter what the volume or what the time. Just make sure the units of time match.

EXERCISE 16.1 MILLILITERS PER HOUR TO DROPS PER MINUTE

(Answers may be found in Appendix D.)

1. You are in the emergency center and the doctor orders an infusion of D$_5$W to run at 200 mL/hr. You have a macrodrip administration set (15 gtt/mL). At how many drops per minute will you set the administration set to drip?

2. Your macrodrip set is 10 gtt/mL. Using problem 1, at how many drops per minute will you set the administration set to drip?

3. The order reads "I.V., N.S., t.r.a. 100 mL/hr." Using a microdrip administration set, at how many drops per minute will you set the administration set to drip?

4. Your macrodrip set is 10 gtt/mL. Using problem 3, at how many drops per minute will you set the administration set to drip?

5. The order reads "I.V., N.S., t.r.a. 250 mL/hr." Using a microdrip administration set, at how many drops per minute will you set the administration set to drip?

6. Your macrodrip set is 10 gtt/mL. Using problem 5, at how many drops per minute will you set the administration set to drip?

7. The order reads "I.V., D_5W, t.r.a. 75 mL/hr." Using a microdrip administration set, at how many drops per minute will you set the administration set to drip?

8. Your macrodrip set is 15 gtt/mL. Using problem 7, at how many drops per minute will you set the administration set to drip?

9. Your macrodrip set is 10 gtt/mL. Using problem 8, at how many drops per minute will you set the administration set to drip?

10. The order in the emergency center reads "I.V., N.S., t.r.a. 350 mL/hr." Using a macrodrip administration set (10 gtt/mL), at how many drops per minute will you set the administration set to drip?

11. You are ordered to administer 1000 milliliters D_5W over the next eight hours. You have a 60 gtt/mL administration set. At how many drops per minute will you set your administration set to drip?

12. You are ordered to administer 10 milliliters of medication over 20 minutes using a microdrip infusion set. At how many drops per minute will you set the administration set to drip?

13. A 6-week-old pediatric patient is admitted to the emergency center severely dehydrated. The orders read to infuse 100 milliliters of 0.45% sodium chloride in 2.5% D_5W over one hour to be followed by 200 milliliters of the same fluid over eight hours. What are the two drip rates using a microdrip set?

14. You have a drip rate to set at 60 gtt/min. To set the drip rate, how many drops should fall in 15 seconds? In 10 seconds? In 5 seconds?

15. You have a drip rate to set at 30 gtt/min. To set the drip rate, how many drops should fall in 15 seconds? In 10 seconds? In 5 seconds?

16.   You have a drip rate to set at 15 gtt/min. To set the drip rate, how many drops should fall in 15 seconds? In 10 seconds? In 5 seconds?

17.   You have a drip rate to set at 120 gtt/min. To set the drip rate, how many drops should fall in 15 seconds? In 10 seconds? In 5 seconds?

18.   The order on the patient's chart in a busy emergency center reads "1500 mL Plasmanate I.V. over 10 hours." The administration set is a 15 gtt/mL set. At how many drops per minute will you set the administration set to drip?

19.   A few hours later another patient comes into the busy emergency center. The order on that chart reads "Plasmanate I.V. t.r.a. 150 mL/hr." The patient's I.V. has 15 gtt/mL administration set. At how many drops per minute will you set the administration set to drip?

20.   The standing order for stable trauma patients is "N.S. t.r.a. 90 mL/hr" using a 10 gtt/mL administration set. At how many drops per minute will you set the administration set to drip?

Posttest

Directions: Answer the following multiple choice questions. Choose the best answer. For answers, see Appendix E.

1. A mathematical representation for parts of a whole is known as a:

    a. denominator
    b. fraction
    c. numerator
    d. none of the above

2. Fractions can be expressed in many ways. When a fraction is expressed in the form of a numerator and denominator, each as a whole number, it is called a:

    a. common fraction
    b. complex fraction
    c. ratio and proportion
    d. percent

3. The bottom number in a fraction that represents the total number of equal parts in the whole is known as the:

    a. denominator
    b. fraction
    c. numerator
    d. none of the above

4. The top number that represents the number of parts that are being considered is known as the:

    a. denominator
    b. fraction
    c. numerator
    d. none of the above

5. When more than one whole is being considered, it can be expressed as a (an):

    a. numerator
    b. proper fraction
    c. improper fraction
    d. denominator

6. Another way to express parts of a whole is based on multiples of 10. What are those fractions called?

    a. common fraction
    b. complex fraction
    c. ratio and proportion
    d. decimal fractions

7. In the number 123.456, the number 2 is in what place?

    a. hundreds
    b. tens
    c. tenths
    d. hundredths

8. When expressing or documenting decimal fractions that do not have an associated whole number, a zero must always be documented or stated before the decimal.

    a. True
    b. False

9. The comparison of two numbers that are separated by a colon and are somehow related to one another is known as a:

    a. common fraction
    b. ratio
    c. proportion
    d. decimal fraction

10. Two related ratios that are equal can be separated by a double colon and called a:

    a. common fraction
    b. ratio
    c. proportion
    d. decimal fraction

11. The numbers in the middle of a proportion are called the:

    a. extremes
    b. means
    c. mediums
    d. pars

12. Solving for *X* in a proportion and solving for *X* using cross-multiplication with common fractions is mathematically the same thing.

    a. True
    b. False

13. A homogeneous mixture of two or more substances is called a:

    a. solute
    b. heterogeneous
    c. concentration
    d. solution

14. The most common way to express percentage concentrations and that expresses the number of grams in a total volume of 100 milliliters of solution is called a:

    a. weight/weight percent
    b. volume/volume percent
    c. weight/volume percent
    d. none of the above

15. The United States gives the _____ the power to set the standard for weights and measures in the United States.

    a. president
    b. Congress
    c. Omnibus Trade Act
    d. General Conference on Weights and Measures

16. Commonly practiced systems of measurement are also known as:

    a. Babylonian systems
    b. metric systems
    c. Roman systems
    d. customary systems

17. The metric system originated in:

    a. the United States
    b. England
    c. France
    d. Spain

18. Choose the correct abbreviation for milliliters:

    a. ML
    b. ml
    c. mL.
    d. mL

19. Spaces, not commas, are used when writing metric values containing five or more digits.
    a. True
    b. False

20. Convert 55 pounds to kilograms:
    a. 27.5 kg
    b. 24.75 kg
    c. 121 kg
    d. 110 kg

21. Convert 1600 micrograms to milligrams:
    a. 1.6 mg
    b. 1 600 000 mg
    c. 160 mg
    d. 0.16 mg

22. One cubic centimeter or 1 cc is equal to how many milliliters?
    a. 1000 mL
    b. 500 mL
    c. 0.5 mL
    d. 1 mL

23. Convert 1000 milligrams to grams:
    a. 1 g
    b. 10 g
    c. 100 g
    d. 0.1 g

24. An 80-kilogram patient weighs how many pounds?
    a. 160 lb
    b. 40 lb
    c. 36 lb
    d. 176 lb

25. One grain (1 gr) equals how many milligrams?
    a. 32.5 mg
    b. 65 mg
    c. 100 mg
    d. 1 mg

26. Your patient is a known congestive heart failure patient with very "wet and noisy" lung fields and shortness of breath. Medical Control orders 40 milligrams of furosemide I.V. The vial reads "10 mg/mL." How many milliliters will you administer?
    a. 2 mL
    b. 4 mL
    c. 40 mL
    d. 400 mL

27. Your patient has symptomatic bradycardia and meets the criteria for the standing order of 0.5 milligrams of atropine I.V. It comes supplied in your ambulance as 1 mg/10 mL. How many will you give?

    a. 1 mL
    b. 10 mL
    c. 0.5 mL
    d. 5 mL

28. Syrup of ipecac is indicated in an adult overdose patient. There are several vials of the medication each reading "15 mL" in the medicine box. Your standing orders read 15 mL p.o. (by mouth) followed by 1 glass of water for pediatric patients and 30 mL p.o. followed by 1–2 glasses of water for adult patients. How many vials will you administer?

    a. 1 vial
    b. 2 vials
    c. 4 vials
    d. 0.5 vial

29. A patient in mild anaphylaxis needs 75 milligrams of diphenhydramine. The prefilled syringe reads 100 mg/5 mL. How many milliliters will you administer?

    a. 0.4 mL
    b. 3.75 mL
    c. 37.5 mL
    d. 150 mL

30. Your 88-pound patient is experiencing multifocal premature ventricular contractions (P.V.C.s) and complains of chest pain. Your standing orders state to administer 1 mg/kg of lidocaine. The lidocaine in your ambulance reads "100 mg/5 mL." How many milliliters will be administered?

    a. 2 mL
    b. 20 mL
    c. 40 mL
    d. none of the above

31. You are in charge of medication administration at a full arrest. The husband states that the patient weighs about 350 pounds. The senior medic calls for the initial dose of epinephrine. Standing orders call for 0.01 mg/kg initial dose of epinephrine 1:10 000. The prefilled syringe label states 0.1 mg/mL. How many total milliliters of epinephrine will you administer to the patient? (Round to the nearest tenth if necessary.)

    a. 0.16 mL
    b. 16 mL
    c. 20 mL
    d. 35 mL

32. Medical Control has standing orders for 1 g of lidocaine to be added to 250-milliliter bags for all lidocaine I.V. drips. What is the concentration in the bag?

    a. 2 mg/mL
    b. 4 mg/mL
    c. 4 g/mL
    d. 8 mg/mL

33. 200 milligrams of dopamine have been added to a 250-milliliter bag of normal saline. What is the concentration in the bag?

    a. 1600 μg/mL
    b. 800 μg/mL
    c. 400 μg/mL
    d. 200 μg/mL

34. 400 milligrams of dopamine have been added to a 250-milliliter bag of normal saline. What is the concentration in the bag?

    a. 1600 μg/mL
    b. 800 μg/mL
    c. 400 μg/mL
    d. 200 μg/mL

35. There is a prefilled syringe of 2% lidocaine in your ambulance. It contains 5 milliliters. How many milligrams does it contain?

    a. 50 mg
    b. 75 mg
    c. 100 mg
    d. 2 g

36. You are ordered to administer lidocaine in an I.V. drip at 2 mg/min. You have 1 gram of lidocaine to add to a 250-milliliter bag. Using a microdrip administration set (60 gtt/mL), at what rate will you set your administration set to drip?

    a. 15 gtt/min
    b. 30 gtt/min
    c. 45 gtt/min
    d. 60 gtt/min

37. Your patient's blood pressure is critically low following conversion from ventricular fibrillation. Medical Control orders you to mix 200 milligrams of dopamine into a 250-milliliter bag of D$_5$W and infuse it at 400 μg/min. With your microdrip administration set (60 gtt/mL), at what rate will you infuse the solution?

    a. 15 gtt/min
    b. 25 gtt/min
    c. 30 gtt/min
    d. 60 gtt/min

38. An order is received to administer dopamine to a 178-pound patient by mixing 400 milligrams of dopamine into a 250-milliliter bag of D_5W. Dopamine is supplied in ampules containing 200 mg/5 mL. The order is to deliver to the dopamine at 5 μg/kg/min. At how many drops per minute will you adjust your microdrip administration set to drip?

    a. 15 gtt/min
    b. 30 gtt/min
    c. 45 gtt/min
    d. 60 gtt/min

39. You are completing your report after delivering a patient to the emergency room and you notice that the dopamine dose ordered by medical control is missing. To avoid any possible reprimands, you decide to determine the ordered dose based on the information available. The patient weighs 178 pounds, and the I.V. infusion is flowing through a microdrip administration set at 30 gtt/min. The label on the 500-milliliter bag of D_5W reads "800 mg of dopamine added." What was the original dose per kilogram per minute ordered?

    a. 5 μg/kg/min
    b. 10 μg/kg/min
    c. 15 μg/kg/min
    d. 20 μg/kg/min

40. The doctor orders you to start an I.V. of normal saline to run at (t.r.a.) 100 milliliters per hour (100 mL/hr). You have a macrodrip set that delivers 15 drops per 1 milliliter (15 gtt/mL). At how many drops per minute will you set your administration set to drip?

    a. 25 gtt/min
    b. 30 gtt/min
    c. 35 gtt/min
    d. 45 gtt/min

41. A 34-pound pediatric patient in asystole requires 0.02 mg/kg of atropine sulfate. Atropine comes supplied for pediatrics in 0.5 mg/mL prefilled syringes. How many milligrams will you administer?

    a. 0.3 mg
    b. 3 mg
    c. 0.1 mg
    d. 0.7 mg

42. From question 41, how many milliliters will you administer?

    a. 0.5 mL
    b. 0.6 mL
    c. 1 mL
    d. 1.4 mL

43. Your approximately 200-pound patient has converted from V-Fib. Her blood pressure is extremely low. Standing orders call for 5 μg/kg of dopamine hydrochloride (Intropin) per minute. What is the dose per minute to be administered to this patient?

    a. 4.5 mg/min
    b. 450 mg/min
    c. 450 μg/min
    d. 1000 μg/min

44. A 50-year-old female patient in cardiac arrest shows V-Fib on the monitor. The V-Fib has been refractory to other treatments and the doctor orders 300 mg slow I.V. of amiodarone (Cordarone). It comes supplied in ampules of 50 mg/mL (3 mL total). How many milliliters will you administer?

    a. 3 mL
    b. 6 mL
    c. 1 mL
    d. 12 mL

45. A patient with chronic back pain is being prepared for a long transport. Protocols allow for 15 mg ketorolac (Toradol) to be administered I.V. It comes supplied in a 2 mL prefilled syringe labeled 30 mg/mL. How many milliliters will you administer?

    a. 1 mL
    b. 2 mL
    c. 15 mL
    d. 30 mL

46. Your patient is a 19-year-old with severe asthma. Terbutaline (Brethine) 0.25 mg subcutaneous is part of the standing orders. It comes supplied in 1 mg/mL ampules. How many milliliters will you administer?

    a. 1 mL
    b. 0.25 mL
    c. 10 mL
    d. 0.5 mL

47. As one part of the Nontraumatic Chest Pain protocol, you may administer morphine sulfate in 2 mg increments every 5–10 minutes up to a maximum of 10 mg. The vial in your unit reads "10 mg/1 mL." How many milliliters will you administer for your first dose?

    a. 0.1 mL
    b. 0.2 mL
    c. 1 mL
    d. 2 mL

48. You are ordered to administer a lidocaine drip at 4 mg/min in a postar-rest patient. The vial supplied in the drug box reads, "1 % lidocaine, 5 g/20 mL." Your supervisor instructs you to add 2 grams of lidocaine to a 250 mL bag. What is the concentration in the bag?

    a. 2 mg/mL
    b. 4 mg/mL
    c. 8 mg/mL
    d. 16 mg/mL

49. From problem 48, using a microdrip administration set, at what rate will you set it to drip?

    a. 10 gtt/min
    b. 15 gtt/min
    c. 30 gtt/min
    d. 60 gtt/min

50. You have a manual drip rate to set at 30 gtt/min. From the choices below, which is the correct setting?

    a. 1 drop should fall each second
    b. 1 drop should fall every other second
    c. 2 drops should fall each second
    d. none of the above

APPENDICES

The answers to the pretest, posttest, and exercises are provided in this section. Having your answers and work in a notebook helps when you refer to this section. If you have questions, refer first to the chapter that you are working from. If you are still having problems, ask your instructor.

Oh, don't the days seem lank and long
When all goes right and nothing goes wrong,
And isn't your life extremely flat
With nothing whatever to grumble at!
—W.S. Gilbert—

PRETEST ANSWER KEY

(To find out how to solve a problem, a chapter (or section) reference is provided after each answer.)

1. 3 (Section 1.1)

2. 7 (Section 1.1)

3. 1 (Section 1.1)

4. 9 (Section 1.1)

5. complex fraction (Section 1.1)

6. proper fraction (Section 1.1)

7. improper fraction (Section 1.1)

8. $\frac{5}{4}$ (Section 1.1)

9. $\frac{65}{6}$ (Section 1.1)

10. $3\frac{1}{4}$ (Section 1.1)

11. $10\frac{7}{9}$ (Section 1.1)

12. equal (Section 1.1)

13. not equal (Section 1.1)

14. $1\frac{19}{126}$ (Section 1.2)

15. $12\frac{41}{45}$ (Section 1.2)

16. $\frac{1}{24}$ (Section 1.3)

17. $\frac{11}{12}$ (Section 1.3)

18. $3\frac{3}{8}$ (Section 1.4)

19. $\frac{1}{84}$ (Section 1.4)

20. $\frac{3}{200}$ (Section 1.5)

21. $2713\frac{1}{2}$ (Section 1.5)

22. 43.95 (Section 2.2)

23. 7.06 (7.0561) (Section 2.2)

24. 1.55 (Section 2.3)

25. 0.81 (0.813) (Section 2.3)

26. 5.63 (5.625) (Section 2.4)

27. 0.03 (0.029766) (Section 2.4)

28. 28.57 (28.571428. . .) (Section 2.5)

29. 0.19 (0.189393. . .) (Section 2.5)

30. 3 : 20 (Chapter 3)

31. $\frac{3}{1}$ (Chapter 3)

32. 18 (Chapter 3)

33. 18 (Chapter 3)

34. 25 (Section 4.2)

35. 0.18 (Section 4.2)

36. 250 (Section 4.2)

37. 0.67 (0.66. . .) (Chapter 5)

38. $\frac{1}{4}$ (Chapter 5)

39. 45% (Chapter 5)

40. $\frac{11}{20}$ (Chapter 5)

ANSWERS TO SECTION ONE EXERCISES

EXERCISE 1.1

1. 2
2. 5
3. 17
4. 2
5. 4
6. 5
7. 8
8. 35
9. 11
10. 2
11. improper
12. proper
13. proper
14. improper
15. proper
16. $2\frac{1}{3}$
17. $3\frac{1}{6}$
18. $6\frac{1}{2}$
19. $9\frac{1}{2}$
20. $2\frac{7}{9}$
21. $\frac{3}{2}$
22. $\frac{7}{3}$
23. $\frac{97}{6}$
24. $\frac{100}{3}$

25. $\frac{47}{5}$
26. $\frac{1}{4}$
27. $\frac{4}{5}$
28. $\frac{1}{10}$
29. $\frac{1}{4}$
30. $\frac{2}{3}$
31. $\frac{4}{12}, \frac{3}{12}, \frac{6}{12}$
32. $\frac{8}{16}, \frac{2}{16}, \frac{1}{16}$
33. $\frac{9}{18}, \frac{12}{18}, \frac{15}{18}, \frac{14}{18}$
34. $\frac{230}{240}, \frac{75}{240}, \frac{222}{240}$
35. $\frac{8}{72}, \frac{33}{72}, \frac{28}{72}$
36. equal
37. equal
38. not equal
39. equal
40. not equal

EXERCISE 1.2

1. $\frac{3}{5}$
2. $\frac{5}{6}$
3. $1\frac{1}{24}$
4. $4\frac{1}{3}$
5. $2\frac{1}{4}$
6. $5\frac{1}{2}$
7. 3
8. $8\frac{1}{4}$

ANSWERS TO SECTION ONE EXERCISES (cont.)

9. $3\frac{7}{9}$

10. $12\frac{41}{45}$

11. $11\frac{19}{24}$

12. $\frac{65}{72}$

13. $6\frac{7}{30}$

14. $9\frac{37}{84}$

15. $7\frac{5}{24}$

EXERCISE 1.3

1. $\frac{1}{2}$

2. $\frac{1}{24}$

3. $\frac{1}{48}$

4. $\frac{11}{12}$

5. $4\frac{5}{6}$

6. $4\frac{3}{4}$

7. $1\frac{17}{24}$

8. $2\frac{7}{10}$

9. $66\frac{23}{33}$

10. $75\frac{1}{100}$

EXERCISE 1.4

1. $\frac{1}{4}$

2. $\frac{1}{6}$

3. $\frac{1}{96}$

4. $\frac{1}{8}$

5. $3\frac{3}{8}$

6. $1\frac{1}{9}$

7. 12

8. $\frac{31}{48}$

9. $\frac{1}{24}$

10. $\frac{5}{96}$

11. 2

12. 405

13. 1500

14. 30

15. 60

16. 60

17. 25

18. 200

19. 60

20. 30

EXERCISE 1.5

1. $\frac{1}{2}$

2. $\frac{1}{2}$

3. $\frac{1}{300}$

4. $\frac{3}{200}$

5. $\frac{1}{30}$

6. $\frac{3}{20}$

7. $\frac{1}{100}$

8. $3\frac{1}{3}$

9. $3\frac{1}{2}$

10. 1206

ANSWERS TO SECTION ONE EXERCISES (cont.)

CHAPTER 1 TEST: COMMON FRACTIONS

1. fraction

2. denominator

3. numerator

4. proper

5. improper

6. 1 or one

7. 1 or one

8. prime

9. lowest

10. common

11. $\frac{2}{5}$

12. $\frac{35}{72}$

13. $\frac{1}{2}$

14. $\frac{3}{10}$

15. 1500

16. 120

17. 180

18. $\frac{3}{20}$

19. $\frac{1}{300}$

20. $\frac{1}{30}$

EXERCISE 2.1

1. thousandths

2. thousands

3. ones

4. ten thousandths

5. hundredths

6. tenths

7. tens

8. hundredths

9. hundredths

10. ones

11. 25.33

12. 36.01

13. 50.35

14. 1723.4

15. 0.01

16. 25.4

17. 100.5

18. 75.2

19. 10

20. 10

EXERCISE 2.2

1. 28

2. 43.95

3. 26.58 (26.575)

4. 2.76

5. 74.03

6. 13.22

7. 25.84 (25.839)

ANSWERS TO SECTION ONE EXERCISES (cont.)

8. 7.06 (7.0561)

9. 10.12

10. 9.55

EXERCISE 2.3

1. 749.5

2. 7.1

3. 2.74

4. 0.91

5. 374.25

6. 0.25

7. 32.8

8. 3.8

9. 1.55

10. 3.28

11. 0.9

12. 0.5

13. 0.3

14. 2.5

15. 1.5

EXERCISE 2.4

1. 3

2. 0.31 (0.3125)

3. 3

4. 11.7

5. 2.06 (2.0625)

6. 0.16 (0.1587)

7. 64.82

8. 250.6 (250.60086)

9. 0.03 (0.029766)

10. 0.1 (0.09795)

11. 45

12. 90

13. 150

14. 10

15. 1

EXERCISE 2.5

1. 28.57 (28.5714. . .)

2. 10.33 (10.333. . .)

3. 8.54 (8.5416. . .)

4. 2825

5. 2500

6. 10.09 (10.0909. . .)

7. 5

8. 40.06

9. 2.24 (2.2388. . .)

10. 0.004 (0.00433. . .)

CHAPTER 2 TEST: DECIMAL FRACTIONS

1. decimal point

2. tenths

3. hundredths

ANSWERS TO SECTION ONE EXERCISES (cont.)

4. zero
5. rounding off
6. 50.5
7. 10
8. 10
9. 22.222
10. 0.9
11. 0.5
12. 0.9
13. 2.5
14. 0.5
15. 99
16. 45
17. 1
18. 10.09
19. 220
20. 20

EXERCISE 3.1

1. 1:10
2. 4:5
3. 200:10
4. 100:5
5. 500:10
6. $\frac{1}{2}$
7. $\frac{1}{250}$

8. $\frac{8}{5}$
9. $\frac{10}{1}$
10. $\frac{3}{1}$
11. 1 and 10
12. 100 and 0.5
13. 40 and 5
14. 2 and 5
15. 10 and 100
16. 2 and 5
17. 5 and 10
18. 10 and 20
19. 1 and 10
20. 1000 and 1

EXERCISE 3.2

1. 1
2. 12
3. 5
4. 100
5. 18
6. 100
7. 1
8. 3
9. 4
10. 4
11. 1
12. 5

ANSWERS TO SECTION ONE EXERCISES (cont.)

13. 0.75

14. 75

15. 5

16. 1

17. 10

18. 0.8

19. 6

20. 5

CHAPTER 3 TEST: RATIOS AND PROPORTIONS

1. ratio

2. colon

3. proportion

4. double colon

5. extremes

6. 1

7. 1

8. 2

9. 4

10. 0.8

EXERCISE 4.1

1. a

2. b

3. c

4. a

5. a

6. true

EXERCISE 4.2

1. 12.5

2. 5%

3. 50

4. 120

5. 5%

6. 80

7. 202.5

8. 80%

9. 200

10. 5%

EXERCISE 5.1

PERCENTAGE	DECIMAL	FRACTION	RATIO
1%	0.01	1/100	1:100
3%	0.03	3/100	3:100
5%	0.05	1/20	1:20
10%	0.1	1/10	1:10
12.5%	0.125	1/8	1:8
25%	0.25	1/4	1:4
33%	0.33	1/3	1:3
75%	0.75	3/4	3:4
100%	1.0	1/1	1:1
2.5%	0.025	1/40	1:40
0.125%	0.00125	1/800	1:800

ANSWERS TO SECTION TWO EXERCISES

EXERCISE 6.1

1. b
2. a
3. b
4. d
5. b
6. c
7. b
8. a
9. b
10. b
11. c
12. b
13. d

EXERCISE 6.1 (CONT.)

14. d
15. b

EXERCISE 7.1

1. iv
2. vi
3. ix
4. vii
5. xxx or XXX
6. 2
7. 4
8. 9
9. 19

EXERCISE 7.1 (CONT.)

10. 24

11. fl pt I (1) = ℥ $\overline{xvi}$ or 16 = ℥ $\underline{CXXviii\ or\ 128}$

12. fl ℥ LXiv (64) = ℥ $\underline{viii\ or\ 8}$ = fl pt $\frac{1}{2}$ or $\overline{ss}$

13. gr LX (60) = Э $\underline{iii\ or\ 3}$ = ℥ $\underline{i\ or\ 1}$

14. ℔ 240 = Э $\underline{iv\ or\ 4}$ = ℥ $\frac{1}{2}$ or $\overline{ss}$

15. ℥ XCvi (96) = ℥ $\underline{xii\ or\ 12}$ = lb ap $\underline{i\ or\ 1}$

16. 1 lb ap = gr ap $\underline{5760}$

17. 1 lb avdp = gr avpd $\underline{7000}$

18. 1 lb ap = oz ap $\underline{12}$

19. 1 lb avpd = oz avpd $\underline{16}$

20. 1 tbsp = $\underline{3\ tsp}$

Appendices

149

ANSWERS TO SECTION TWO EXERCISES (cont.)

EXERCISE 8.1

1.	1 g	=	1000 mg
2.	1 mg	=	1000 μg
3.	7 500 mg	=	7.5 g
4.	1 600 μg	=	1.6 mg
5.	1 000 mg	=	1 g
6.	0.75 g	=	750 mg
7.	500 mL	=	0.5 L
8.	0.25 L	=	250 mL
9.	1.6 mg	=	1600 μg
10.	2 500 g	=	2.5 kg
11.	0.715 g	=	715 mg
12.	400 000 μg	=	400 mg
13.	125 mg	=	0.125 g
14.	0.1 g	=	100 mg
15.	0.45 L	=	450 mL
16.	1.5 L	=	1500 mL
17.	80 000 g	=	80 kg
18.	4 000 mg	=	4 g
19.	800 μg	=	0.8 mg
20.	1000 mL	=	1 L
21.	0.8 mg	=	800 μg
22.	250 mL	=	0.25 L
23.	75 000 g	=	75 kg
24.	400 μg	=	0.4 mg

25.	200 mg	=	200 000 μg
26.	1 000 mg	=	1 000 000 μg
27.	0.000 5 g	=	0.5 mg
28.	10 kg	=	10 000 000 mg
29.	0.0016 kg	=	1600 mg
30.	0.03 L	=	30 mL
31.	200 000 μg	=	200 mg
32.	1 000 g	=	1 kg
33.	600 μg	=	0.6 mg
34.	10 000 mg	=	10 g
35.	4 mg	=	0.004 g
36.	6.8 kg	=	6800 g
37.	1 600 μg	=	1.6 mg
38.	0.001 6 g	=	1600 μg
39.	1 500 mL	=	1.5 L
40.	1 μg	=	0.001 mg

EXERCISE 9.1

1.	$\frac{1}{4}$ gr	=	16.25 mg
2.	55 lb	=	24.75 kg
3.	45 mL	=	1.5 oz
4.	12 mL	=	2.4 tsp
5.	16.25 mg	=	$\frac{1}{4}$ gr
6.	12 oz	=	360 mL
7.	500 mL	=	0.52 qt
8.	45 mL	=	$1\frac{1}{2}$ oz

ANSWERS TO SECTION TWO EXERCISES (cont.)

9.	2 tbsp	=	30 mL		33.	90 mL	=	3 oz
10.	1 tbsp	=	15 mL		34.	10 mL	=	10 cc
11.	$\frac{1}{2}$ gr	=	32.5 mg		35.	2 tsp	=	10 mL
12.	1 g	=	15 gr		36.	2 qt	=	1900 mL
13.	gr $\overline{\text{iss}}$	=	97.5 mg		37.	500 mL	=	0.5 L
14.	4 mL	=	0.133 oz		38.	gr vii$\overline{\text{ss}}$	=	0.4875 g (0.5 g)
15.	3 oz	=	90 mL		39.	gr xx	=	1.3 g
16.	180 lb	=	81 kg		40.	220 lb	=	99 kg
17.	$\frac{1}{6}$ gr	=	10.8 mg		41.	5 gr	=	0.33 g
18.	150 lb	=	67.5 kg		42.	88 lb	=	39.6 kg
19.	260 mg	=	4 gr		43.	3 gr	=	195 mg
20.	5.85 g	=	90 gr		44.	80 kg	=	177.78 lb
21.	7 lb	=	3.15 kg		45.	50 lb	=	22.5 kg
22.	3 oz	=	90 mL		46.	356 lb	=	160.2 kg
23.	11 lb	=	4.95 kg		47.	75 gr	=	4.9 g
24.	2 tbsp	=	30 mL		48.	90 kg	=	200 lb
25.	200 lb	=	90 kg		49.	30 mL	=	2 tbsp
26.	0.05 g	=	0.75 or $\frac{3}{4}$ gr		50.	80 lb	=	36 kg
27.	0.3 mL	=	0.01 oz					
28.	$\frac{1}{2}$ gr	=	32.5 mg					
29.	$1\frac{1}{2}$ gr	=	97.5 mg					
30.	30 kg	=	66.7 lb					
31.	1000 mL	=	2.08 pt					
32.	2000 mL	=	2.114 qt					

ANSWERS TO SECTION THREE EXERCISES

EXERCISE 10.1

1. 10 mL
2. 4 mL
3. 5 mL
4. 100 mL
5. 2 mL
6. 0.33 mL (leading zero required)
7. 1.5 mL
8. 2 tablets
9. 4 mL
10. 0.5 mL (leading zero required)
11. 0.75 mL (leading zero required)
12. 0.75 mL(leading zero required)
13. 2 mL
14. 4 mL
15. 2.5 mL
16. 8 mL
17. 1 mL
18. 30 mL
19. 50 mL
20. 5 mL
21. 2 tabs
22. 5 mL
23. 3.75 mL
24. 2400–3200 mg

25. 50 mg
26. 0.8 mL (leading zero required)
27. 270 μg
28. 6 mL
29. 5 mL
30. 0.3 mL (leading zero required)
31. 0.5 mL (leading zero required)
32. 1.2 mg
33. 0.5 mL (leading zero required)
34. a. 4 mL   b. 2 vials
35. 0.5 mL (leading zero required)
36. 4 mL
37. 0.25 mL (leading zero required)
38. 0.2 mL (leading zero required)
39. 10 mL
40. 2.5 mL

EXERCISE 11.1

1. a. 67.5 mg   b. 3.4 mL
2. a. 337.5 mg   b. 6.8 mL
3. a. 1.3 mg   b. 0.6 mL (leading zero required)
4. a. 72 mEq   b. 72 mL
5. a. 0.2 mg (leading zero required)
   b. 0.2 mL (leading zero required)
6. a. 0.6 mg (leading zero required)
   b. 0.2 mL (leading zero required)

ANSWERS TO SECTION THREE EXERCISES (cont.)

7. a. 1.2 mg   b. 0.4 mL (leading zero required)

8. a. 0.2 mg   b. 0.4 mL

9. a. 22.5 mg   b. 45 mL

10. a. 40.5 mg   b. 0.8 mL

11. 500 mg/min

12. a. 16.2 mg   b. 16.2 mL

13. a. 1.1 mg   b. 11 mL

14. a. 35.1 mg   b. 17.6 mL

15. a. 175.5 mg   b. 8.8 mL   c. 2 vials

16. a. 11.7 mg   b. 11.7 mL   c. two (One vial contains 10 mg and 12 mg is needed. Therefore, 2 mL from a second vial are needed to complete the ordered dose.)

17. a. 40 mg   b. 4 mL   c. 2 vials

18. a. 112.7 mg   b. 5.6 mL

19. a. 2.5 mg   b. 0.25 mL

20. a. 49.5 mEq   b. 49.5 mL

EXERCISE 12.1

1. b   2. c   3. a

4. c   5. a   6. a

7. true

EXERCISE 12.2

1. a. 3 g   b. Dilute the 50% dextrose with equal amounts of water or normal saline.   c. 12 mL

2. a. 4 g   b. Dilute the 50% dextrose with equal amounts of water or normal saline.   c. 16 mL

3. 0.01 mg/kg

4. 0.5 mg

5. 64 mL

6. 1 : 10 000

7. 9 mL

8. 1 : 1000

9. a. 2 g   b. Expel all but 10 mL and refill with sterile water or normal saline.   c. 20 mL

EXERCISE 13.1

1. 800 μg/mL

2. 9 g

3. 5 mg/mL

4. 5 mL

5. 4 μg/mL

6. 50 mg

7. 100 mg

8. 4 mg/mL

9. 25 g

10. 20 mg/mL

11. 2.25 g

12. 4 mg/mL

13. 10 mg/mL

14. 5 mg/mL

15. 1600 μg/mL

16. 4 μg/mL

ANSWERS TO SECTION THREE EXERCISES (cont.)

17. 3.75 mL

18. 3 mL

19. 800 μg/mL

20. 10 μg/mL

EXERCISE 14

1. 60 gtt/min

2. 10 gtt/min

3. 30 gtt/min

4. 5 gtt/min

5. 30 gtt/min

6. 15 gtt/min

7. 4 gtt/min

8. 45 gtt/min

9. 45 gtt/min

10. 120 gtt/min

11. 30 gtt/min

12. 30 gtt/min

13. 60 gtt/min

14. 10 gtt/min

15. 30 gtt/min

16. 5 gtt/min

17. 30 gtt/min

18. 15 gtt/min

19. 23 gtt/min

20. 6 gtt/min

21. 30 gtt/min

22. 100 gtt/min

EXERCISE 15

1. 30 gtt/min

2. 15 gtt/min

3. 30 gtt/min

4. 45 gtt/min

5. 45 gtt/min

6. 90 gtt/min

7. 10 μg/kg/min

8. 4 μg/kg/min

9. 15 gtt/min

10. 51–52 gtt/min

EXERCISE 16

1. 50 gtt/min

2. 33 gtt/min

3. 100 gtt/min

4. 17 gtt/min

5. 250 gtt/min

6. 42 gtt/min

7. 75 gtt/min

8. 19 gtt/min

9. 13 gtt/min

10. 58 gtt/min

11. 125 gtt/min

ANSWERS TO SECTION THREE EXERCISES (cont.)

12. 30 gtt/min

13. 100 gtt/min (first hour)
    25 gtt/min (over 8 hours)

14. 15 sec = 15 gtt
    10 sec = 10 gtt
    5 sec = 5 gtt

15. 15 sec = 8 gtt
    10 sec = 5 gtt
    5 sec = 3 gtt

16. 15 sec = 4 gtt
    10 sec = 3 gtt
    5 sec = 1 gtt

17. 15 sec = 30 gtt
    10 sec = 20 gtt
    5 sec = 10 gtt

18. 38 gtt/min

19. 38 gtt/min

20. 15 gtt/min

ANSWERS TO POSTTEST

1. b

2. a

3. a

4. c

5. c

6. d

7. b

8. a

9. b

10. c

11. b

12. a

13. d

14. c

15. b

16. d

17. c

18. d

19. a

20. b

21. a

22. d

23. a

24. d (Hint: kg to lb, not lb to kg.)

25. b

26. b

27. d

28. b

29. b

30. a

31. b

32. b

33. b

34. a

35. c (Hint: What does 2% mean? See Chapter 12.)

36. b

37. c

38. a

39. b (Hint: Work the clock process backward.)

40. a

41. a

42. b

43. c

44. b

45. a

46. b

47. b

48. c

49. c

50. b

CONVERSION FACTORS FORMAT BETWEEN THE U. S. CUSTOMARY SYSTEM AND THE METRIC SYSTEM(APPROXIMATE)

VOLUME

60 μgtt (microdrip)	= 1 mL
macrogtt sets varies*	
1 tsp	= 5 mL
1 tbsp	= 15 mL
1 fl oz	= 30 mL
1 cup	= 240 mL
1 pt	= 480 mL
1 qt	= 950 mL
1 gal	= 3.8 L
1 L	= 1.057 qt

LENGTH

1 in	= 2.54 cm
1 ft	= 30.48 cm
1 yd	= 0.914 m
1 mi	= 1.6 km
1 m	= 39.37 in

WEIGHT

1 gr	= 65 mg
1 oz	= 28.35 g
1 lb	= 453.6 g
1 kg	= 2.2 lb
1 g	= 15 gr

TEMPERATURE CONVERSIONS

To convert Fahrenheit to Celsius:

$$(^\circ F - 32) \times \tfrac{5}{9} = {^\circ}C$$

To convert Celsius to Fahrenheit:

$$(^\circ C \times \tfrac{9}{5}) + 32 = {^\circ}F$$

*Macrodrip administration sets are variable. Check the product label. The most common macrodrip sets are 10 gtt/mL and 15 gtt/mL.

WEIGHT AND TEMPERATURE CONVERSION TABLE

POUNDS	KILOGRAMS	FAHRENHEIT	CELSIUS
5	2.25	0	−17.8
10	4.5	32	0
11.1	5	40	4.4
15	6.75	41	5
20	9	50	10
22.2	10	59	15
25	11.25	60	15.6
30	13.5	68	20
35	15.75	70	21.1
40	18	75	23.9
44.4	20	77	25
45	20.25	80	26.7
50	22.5	85	29.4
55	24.75	86	30
60	27	90	32.2
66.7	30	95	35
70	31.5	**98.6**	**37**
80	36	98	36.7
90	40.5	99	37.2
100	45	100	37.8
111.1	50	101	38.3
120	54	102	38.9
150	67.5	104	40
155.6	70	105	40.5
180	81	106	41.1
200	90	107	41.6
220	99	108	42.2
222.2	100	110	43.3
333.3	150	113	45
350	157.5		
380	171		
400	180		

COMMON RULE OF FOURS CLOCKS

4 mg/mL CLOCK

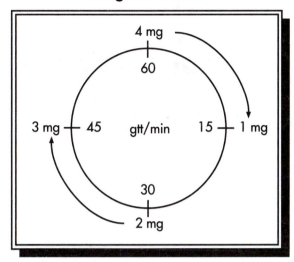

1 gram into 250 milliliters yields 4 mg/mL

4 µg/mL CLOCK

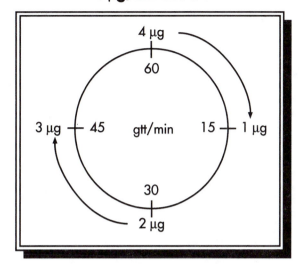

1 milligram into 250 milliliters yields 4 µg/mL

1600 µg/mL CLOCK

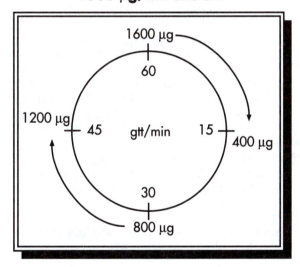

400 milligrams into 250 milliliters yields 1600 µg/mL

800 µg/mL CLOCK

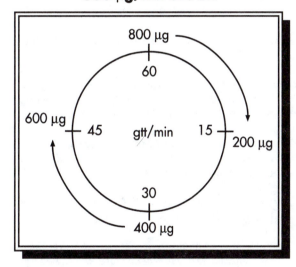

200 milligrams into 250 milliliters yields 800 µg/mL

Bibliography

Biddle, H., and D. Sitler. *Mathematics of Drugs and Solutions*, 6th ed. Philadelphia: Davis, 1963.

Brown, H. *A Father's Book of Wisdom.* Nashville: Rutledge Hill, 1988.

Carver, G. *A Metric America: A Decision Whose Time Has Come–for Real,* NISTIR 4858. Gaithersburg, MD: U.S. Department of Commerce, 1992.

Carver, G. *Metrication: An Economic Wake-up Call for US Industry,* NISTIR 5154. Gaithersburg, MD: U.S. Department of Commerce, 1993.

Curren, A., and L. Munday. *Math for Meds,* 7th ed. San Diego: WI Publications, 1995.

General Services Administration. *Preferred Metric Units for General Use by the Federal Government,* Federal Standard 376A. Washington, DC: The Administration, 1993.

Hegstad, L., and W. Hayek. *Essential Drug Dosage Calculations.* Bowie, MD: Brady, 1983.

James, M., and J. James. *Passion for Life.* New York: Dutton, 1991.

McCoubrey, A. "Measures and Measuring Systems," *Encyclopedia Americana,* Vol. 18, pp. 584–597. Danbury, CT: Grolier, 1987.

National Institute of Standards and Technology, U.S. Department of Commerce, *Interpretation of the SI for the United States and Metric Conversion Policy for Federal Agencies,* NIST Special Publication 814. Gaithersburg, MD: The Administration, 1991.

National Institute of Standards and Technology, U.S. Department of Commerce; *Metric Style Guide for the News Media,* NIST LC 1137. Gaithersburg, MD: The Administration, 1992.

National Institute of Standards and Technology, U.S. Department of Commerce; *The United States and the metric system,* NIST LC 1136. Gaithersburg, MD: The Administration, 1992.

Texas Children's Hospital, *Drug Information and Formulary,* 4th ed.

The Oxford Dictionary of Quotations, 3rd ed., New York: Oxford University Press, 1980.

Remsen, S., and P. Ackermann. *Calculations for the Medical Laboratory.* Boston: Little, Brown, 1977.

Standard Educational Corporation. "Weights and Measures," *New Standards Encyclopedia,* Vol. 17, pp. w124–w126. Chicago: The Corporation, 1983.

Index

161